SARAH KUGLER POWERS

# THE EXCEPTION
## AND THE RULE

*On Being Stage IV*

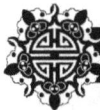

Lucky Bat Books

*For Harrison*
*True love stories never have endings.*

A Lucky Bat Book

The Exception and the Rule: On Being Stage IV

Copyright 2015 by Sarah Kugler Powers

First Printing

Cover Artist:
Danielle Tunstall
http://www.danielletunstall.com
Cover Design:
Nuno Moreira
http://www.nmdesign.org

Published by Lucky Bat Books
LuckyBatBooks.com

10 9 8 7 6 5 4 3 2 1

ISBN: 978-1-939051-98-1

This book also available in digital formats.
Discover other titles by the author at
http://www.sarahkuglerpowers.com

# CONTENTS

# FOREWORD

At the age of twenty-four, Sarah Kugler Powers was given a two-per-cent chance of surviving stage IV cancer. She read how other cancer patients survived overwhelming odds and this helped ignite in her "a small part that refused to believe that the odds were too great to overcome . . ."

When I was thirty-two, I was diagnosed with terminal cancer and given a ten-percent chance to live one year, so I have some idea of the pressure put on this brave young woman to give up control of her treatment and her life to the "experts." Every week during the initial months of my own diagnosis and treatment some expert told me in words and looks that I would soon die, that my questions about treatment alternatives and about my ability to father children were irrelevant and evidence of my refusal to accept the inevitable death sentence. Well, the experts were wrong, and thankfully Sarah and I beat the odds. It doesn't always happen that way, but we are living proof that—with good medical treatment and a stubborn refusal to be completely overwhelmed by statistics—it is possible.

The shock of the diagnosis, the desperate need for help, the difficult medical language and treatment terms, and the authority of the doctor all conspire to pressure the patient to not ask questions but to just fol-low orders. Under such pressure it's all too easy for patients to fall into a passive role, at a crucial time when—as I argue in my *New England Journal of Medicine* article (February 8, 1979) "Fighting Cancer: One Patient's Perspective"—the patient needs to be an active partner on the healthcare team.

Repeatedly, it has been found that patients who actively participate in their healthcare decisions have less stress, improved mood, and generally have better outcomes. In fact, we now know that asking questions, express-ing difficult emotions, and playing an active role in treatment decisions, is simply good medicine that seems to optimize the patient's attitude and chances of survival. To paraphrase Norman Cousins in the foreword to my book, *Coping with the Emotional Impact of Cancer* (Bay Tree Publishing, 2009), being actively involved can serve as an antidote for the feelings of helplessness and loss of control that are so prevalent among patients with cancer.

Patients are inspired by and learn from remarkable stories of survival such as Sarah Kugler Powers', but more than that, they want to know, "How can I do what you did? And how did you do it?" These are very difficult questions to answer because when you're under pressure and fighting for your life you will discover resources deep inside that you didn't know you had. These resources will come to you when you need them most—as they did for me when I heard myself tell my doctor, "Surgery is not scheduled for tomorrow. I haven't had time to talk with my family or to consider a second opinion," in a voice that sounded much stronger and more confident than I felt at that moment.

In an attempt to answer the question, "How did you have the nerve to speak up for yourself with your doctors?" I think back to being raised in Jersey City, NJ, during the time of gangs and bullies and fighting my way back from school to get home or bluffing my way out of a fight. I think back to how I found the courage to speak up in the army to protect my men from being used in Vietnam for some captain's idea of a heroic patrol. I'm reminded of seeing other patients in the hospital waiting room and feeling a deep sense of responsibility to speak up for those who might be less assertive than me.

Like so many cancer patients, I wanted to make my experience and suffering mean something, serve some higher purpose. The cancer had already spread (metastasized) to my left lung, so I knew I could die within a year. But I felt an obligation to spend that year trying to humanize medicine for future patients and for doctors and nurses. I was a Vietnam veteran as well as a new psychologist who was unusually equipped to speak up for patients and to cope with the stress and pressures of a terminal cancer diagnosis.

I had been a paratrooper who learned that even though I didn't want to jump out of an airplane, I could choose to fully commit to leaving that plane in a way that would maximize my chances of survival.

I used that same sense of choice in arguing with my surgeon to receive chemotherapy. The doctors and nurses kept telling me that the chemotherapy was "toxic," but it was my only chance to get rid of the cancer that was rapidly spreading through my blood stream.

In order to take the experimental chemo week after week for more than nine months, I pushed aside the word "toxic" and thought of the chemo as "strong medicine" that kills rapidly dividing cancer cells. Hair cells are also rapidly dividing, as are the cells of the mucous membrane. So losing my hair and getting blisters on my tongue could be thought of as a sign that my strong ally was working to kill cancer.

I was arrogant enough to think that I might be able to improve the quality of medical treatment for cancer patients by demonstrating to my doctors that the mind and emotions have a role to play in adapting to, cooperating with, and contributing to the efficacy of medical treatment. I changed my diet, tripling the amount of vegetables and stopping red meat while my body coped with chemotherapy. I dedicated some time each day for entering a meditative, relaxed state to give energy over to my body and my immune system by lowering my stress hormones.

I can't tell you what you should do, nor can I tell you exactly how I did it, but I can tell you that when you survive against the odds, you are not just two-percent or ten-percent alive, you are one- hundred-percent alive. I can't tell you what to do to increase your chances of survival because your condition and experiences are different from mine, but I can tell you:

I questioned my doctors about alternatives and stayed alert to their biases from their medical/disease-oriented perspective.

I maintained a more positive view of the robustness of the human spirit and body and that the body is active in holding cancer in place, not just allowing cancer to spread.

It was this belief that allowed me to question my surgeon about the wisdom of removing my lung—the lung I argued was filtering my blood and holding on to cancer cells.

I fought to get on an experimental protocol and chose and re-chose chemotherapy when the side effects became more severe.

I had a sense of mission: to make my experience with cancer and medical treatment helpful to others.

And, like Sarah Kugler Powers, I spoke about my experience and wrote about it to reach people like you.

There are several similarities in how Sarah and I coped. Strangely enough we both fought to get chemotherapy, and it was this relatively new, often feared, treatment that contributed to saving our lives. We both had to argue for and discuss alternatives with our doctors, and both of us had to fire our initial doctors before finding doctors who could listen, include us as part of the treatment team, and provide a healing relationship. We both also have told our story in the hope that you, the reader, could benefit from our experience in coping with cancer as part of your therapy team.

Your temperament and style may be different from those of others, but that doesn't make it wrong—nor does it suggest that you must follow our way of coping. There's something very powerful about believing in yourself and speaking your truth and expressing your feelings (especially the more difficult ones such as anger and depression) that lowers stress hormones and improves the strength of your immune system.

Those who are not comfortable questioning their doctors could benefit from the support of patient advocates (perhaps a friend or a medical social worker or a chaplain). One of the reasons people like Sarah have written about their experience is to give a voice to those who are less prepared to speak up for themselves. We know how asserting an opinion by asking, for example, for another PET scan or a second or third opinion can save a life (as it did Sarah's).

Sarah writes wisely about the insidiousness of the language of cancer that communicates a message to our brains and bodies of a "war to be fought" and to be won or lost. This unfortunate language encourages the media and family members to pressure patients to "fight harder" when a more effective approach might be to conserve energy in a meditative state that allows the immune system to do its job in cooperation with medical treatment. As Dr. Lewis Thomas writes in *The Lives of a Cell* (Viking Press, 1975), you don't tell a killer T cell what to do. That is, since the killer T, or immune system "white cells," fight cancer, you would do well to get out of their way and let them work for you rather than wasting valuable resources trying to boss them.

If you are a newly diagnosed cancer patient or a family member in a similar situation, you can take courage from Sarah's remarkable story and book. This is a book I wish I had had when I was first diagnosed with cancer. I highly recommend Sarah Kugler Powers' *The Exception and The Rule* (Lucky Bat Books, 2015).

Neil A. Fiore, PhD, November 18, 2014

# PREFACE

Imagine for a moment that you are about to face the most difficult challenge of your life. You are weak, you are weary, and your spirit is broken. Your opponent is stronger than you, more resilient than you, and just as clever as you. You face overwhelming odds of defeat. In a wager for your life, would you bet on you? At that moment when you turn to face your opponent, are you the exception or are you the rule?

In 2011, in the middle of law school, I found myself in this exact situation. I didn't know it then, but my opponent had been preparing for this day for some time. When I faced my aggressor, I was blindsided. I was told I had one month to live. At the age of twenty-four, I was dying of stage IV cancer.

In the wager for my life, I bet on me.

But I didn't start out willing to do that. Even though I was working toward becoming an attorney and was not the kind of person to believe what anyone said without my own research, when I was first diagnosed, and for months after, I was a passive recipient of medical care. I did what my doctors told me, without question or explanation. It was only when I realized that passivity could kill me (and it almost did) that I began being an active, sometimes even confrontational, participant in my care.

I didn't always agree with my doctors. Sometimes this was because something was obviously missed or plain wrong, but sometimes it was just because I knew they didn't have the same skin in the game I did. I knew the difference.

In this book, I have included transcriptions of recordings of some of my medical appointments. It was important to me to include them verbatim because 1) I have a legal background; I am a natural chronicler, and 2) because they are good examples of some of the most valuable lessons I learned. I wanted to give readers those experiences in their purest form, unchanged by memory loss, chemo brain, or time. Some are from recordings I made of my appointments, but some are from my medical records. Nothing more, nothing less.

Not all of my medical care was... let's say adequate. And though I stand behind everything here, I changed some of the physicians' names in this book because in the end it's just not about them. It's about you, the reader, and using my experience to improve yours.

I was angry for a long time about some of the care I received. But maybe more so, I was angry with myself for being so passive in the beginning. It's not like me (as you might notice from Alan Dershowitz's quote on the back of this book). While there were parts of my personality and history that helped me take on that active role, I had to dig deep to find them in the midst of the whirlwind that is a terminal cancer diagnosis. Everything moved so quickly and with such intricacy and intensity that I could do little more than try to keep up.

No one is born ready for a terminal diagnosis. But once you get it, you best get ready fast, because cancer is not going to slow down and let you catch up. Neither are your doctors.

Since my diagnosis, I have found purpose and grace in walking friends and even strangers through the maelstrom of cancer treatment. I have held the hands of people I love as they slip away. I have let mine be the voice that fought with doctors and insurance companies after for the sake of family left in the aftermath. Maybe I'm practicing for my own "someday," but I refuse to let my experience mean nothing. It took me too long to take back the reins, and I lost too much to that passivity. I'm going to do all I can with the time I have left to make sure others don't do the same.

I suppose I always knew I would write a book at some point in my life. The written word has always been my love, my guide, my way of entering and being in the world. The legal world was a place I could parse even the most nuanced sentence and wring from it every shade of meaning. I loved every minute I was able to spend among thick books and dog-eared briefs. Writing books was something I was going to do when I retired, with a good long life full of a staggering array of experiences from which I could draw.

Never in my wildest dreams did I think *this* would be the book I would write. But writing this book, in spite of how painful it has been at times, may very well be the most important accomplishment of my life. This book has played an instrumental role in my work in the cancer community because there is a real value derived from sharing our stories, even those as dark as mine.

I'm sharing my story in hopes of lighting the way for those of you who will find yourselves embarking on this journey after me. Although this is a path that we all endure alone, we are not without those who have gone before. Neil Fiore lit the way for me; I hope to light the way for you.

I want my words, imperfect as they are, to be a source of companionship to those reaching out in times of great chaos, fear, and uncertainty. Please, reach out. It is the only way to find those of us who are reaching back.

# INTRODUCTION

Every so often, after I wake up in the morning, I find myself staring into the mirror. I am reminded that I am twenty-four years old, and for a brief second I am terrified. It is not my age itself that terrifies me, but rather that my age is no indication of my experience, no tool that can be used to make basic assumptions of who I am, where I have been, nor what lies before me. I have no roadmap, no limitations, and no pre-set guidelines. Everything is possible.

*"You have cancer."*

When I first heard those words, the impact they had shook me like an earthquake. At that moment, my reality crumbled around me. Learning that I had cancer was only the initial tremor, and that was not the end of it. There were aftershocks. My cancer diagnosis was unlike anything else that I had experienced in my life, and the aftershocks came with great force as I learned the specifics of my diagnosis.

Cancer not only shatters the world of the person who is diagnosed, but also the people in that individual's life. The aftershocks are far-reaching and impart damage to each person in an individualized way. The way each of us copes with these developments is unique in many respects, depending upon who we are as individuals. There is no accepted reaction to a cancer diagnosis.

I often hear from physicians, caregivers, patients, and other supporters that no one cancer is the same as another. This statement, which began as a medical fact, has now taken on its own identity as a declaration among many patients and their supporters. They often use this statement as evidence that we as cancer patients cannot be reduced to a number or statistic.

While "there is no right reaction to cancer" is one of my least favorite of the American cancer culture platitudes, it is true nevertheless. I can share with you my experience through firsthand records and stories, but this in no way means that your story will mimic mine. I don't offer my story as a path through the cancer wilderness, but rather as possible signposts along the way. As you go through your own journey (or as you walk with someone else on theirs), I hope what I've been through will save you some time, some effort, and ultimately make your path a little easier.

In sharing my story and the lessons I have learned in my life, I hope that you will find a bit of your story reflected in these pages and that your own story may in part be told as well.

If you are reading this book to better understand what a friend or loved one is going through, please know that I will be as honest as I can. There are a lot of books about cancer and a lot about caregiving, but too many of them hold back on some of the more brutal aspects of the disease in their attempts to alleviate the worry and sensibilities of caregivers. But people with stage IV cancer don't have that luxury.

I wasn't always as understanding of those around me as I wish I were. I didn't always understand what they were going through. I didn't always care. There were times when it was all I could do to survive, and how my cancer was affecting those around me simply was not on my radar. No one is going to make a courageous Lifetime movie of my life. And that's fine.

This book is in three parts because that is how I have come to think of my cancer. There was a beginning, when everything was a shock and an emergency. It was filled with action with little explanation. The diagnosis, the quickness in which action needed to be taken, the just trying to keep up—this was a period of such uncertainty that it felt as if time had stopped. Next came treatment. I think of it as the period when things were being done to me. I shuffled from one doctor to another, one treatment to another, feeling like part of a dance I'd never learned. But eventually it became clear that if I were going to survive, it was going to be up to me to lead. Part three is how I went from passive patient to active participant.

This book is set up so that you can read it beginning to end as a journey, but you can also just flip to the issues with which you may be struggling. Go to the signposts you need, maybe sit and rest there awhile. It's OK. These pages will be here when you're ready.

# PART ONE

## SO IT BEGINS

# CHAPTER ONE

# DIAGNOSIS

*It was the night before my life turned to ash, leaving me an empty shell, a charred remnant of my former self. Cancer would soon strip me of all but my bones, their lovely fragility threatening to splinter under its weight.*

✦

It was November of 2011, and I was nearing the end of my first year of law school at the University of Connecticut. Fall finals were rapidly approaching and fueled almost exclusively by caffeine and Adderall, I spent days leading up to exams tucked away behind my large mahogany desk. I worked steadily, briefing cases, drafting my legendary master outlines, and working voraciously with a sharp precision and diligent work ethic through archives of past years' exams. For days at a time I did not leave my office—apart from short lunch and dinner breaks.

While I pored over the seemingly endless mountain of information, I could not help but notice what had become a familiar pain in my right hip. It had first made itself known a year prior, but it was becoming increasingly difficult to explain away. I was concerned—just not as much as I was concerned about receiving a high score on my law school exams.

The evening before my first exam, I packed up my supplies for the following day, crawled into bed, and snuggled up next to my fiancé, Harrison. I began to fall asleep, listening on my iPad to a law review course, when I was jolted awake by a bolt of searing pain that shot straight through my hip and up my spine. I yelped and threw off the covers, expecting to find blood. For a split second I thought I'd been shot.

This was not the ache I'd been treating with ibuprofen. As I gripped my hip and writhed, Harrison asked what was wrong, what he could do again and again. I felt like I might pass out just from the pain.

When it became clear that there was nothing for Harrison to do to help, he dashed out of the apartment to the nearest pharmacy and bought every type of pain reliever on the shelves.

By the time he returned, less than twenty minutes later, my panic had passed, though the pain had not. It had become a constant roar. As Harrison read labels and shook pills into my hand, we talked about my going to the hospital. Harrison thought I should. But I'd always considered myself too tough for hospitals, and I wasn't going to let a long ER wait make me miss finals. I'd studied too hard. Even after Harrison started to get mad at my stubbornness, I refused to go.

I kept saying it would pass. *Any minute now*, I kept thinking.

I lay in bed for twelve hours, clenching my teeth as I endured the cruel consistency of the pain, all the while thinking it would pass.

It didn't. But I made it through that final. And the next. And the next.

The pain continued almost nightly throughout the two-week final exam period. It would lessen some during the days, enabling me to take tests but robbing me of sleep at night. The pain never was not there—it always was; it was just a matter of the degree. I think it was better during the day because it was mind over matter and when I put my mind to it, I have all-encompassing focus. But at night, when all I could do was lie in bed, there was no escape from the pain. I ate over-the-counter pain killers like candy.

By the evening of December 19, 2011, the pain had subsided enough that I decided not to worry about talking to a doctor until after the holidays. Professor Fischl's contract course, which was by far my favorite, was the last class for which I had an exam. I remember it was raining because I was planning to fly home to our family ranch in Nevada for Christmas break. I was concerned about the runways at the airport and how quickly the rain tended to freeze in the Connecticut winter.

Professor Fischl had told us he would be waiting at a nearby pub following our exam to buy us all a round of drinks to celebrate the end of a successful semester. I had intended to walk over with friends from class. However, it had continued to rain throughout the evening, and the temperature quickly dropped. I decided it would be best to leave directly for the airport to avoid the worsening weather and possibly a flight cancellation.

Following the exam, I wished everyone happy holidays and walked toward my car. I could hear my classmates' laughter echo and fade as a light drizzle fell over the quiet campus. The only other sound was the gentle tumble of the rain mimicking my footsteps. It was peaceful at that moment. As I walked across campus that evening, I was content.

✦

December 20, 2011, began like any other holiday at home. I had spent the day shopping with my mother for Christmas presents for my older brother, younger sister, and father. We laughed about the neighbors and talked about our resolutions for the New Year—how much weight was to be lost and wealth to be acquired—over lunch at one of our favorite restaurants. The day was so simple and set in its tradition. Perhaps that is what made it so quaint and lovely. I enjoyed those afternoons out quite a bit. It was home.

But this was the night before my life turned to ash, leaving me an empty shell, a charred remnant of my former self. Cancer would soon strip me of all but my bones, their lovely fragility threatening to splinter under its weight.

That night, my younger sister, Alyce, drove to the house to stay for a few days—like she did every time I came to visit. She only lived half an hour away, but the ranch was still home, and it was where we all wanted to be for the holidays. She mentioned that I looked unwell, and I asked her if she thought my right leg looked swollen. Alyce was taken aback when I rolled up my pant legs to compare.

"Yes, Sarah, your leg is swollen; you need to tell mom right now," she said.

I agreed, and together we went downstairs and found my mother in the kitchen. I asked her the same question, and instantly she became concerned at the size of my swollen limb. I tried to calm her down and explain to her that it was most likely a blood clot from a lack of exercise and from the long plane ride from Connecticut to Nevada. Nevertheless, the next morning, she called our local family doctor, who urged her to take me to the nearest urgent care facility. In the meantime, Alyce and I conducted Google and WebMD research on unlikely conditions such as elephantitis. As we lightheartedly searched the Internet for possible causes of the swelling, there was an unmistakable fear in the backs of both of our minds that it could be something more serious.

The following morning, December 21, 2011, my mother and I pulled up to the local urgent care. I was dressed casually in a Nike running shirt and fitted sweatpants. The nurse called us into one of the rooms, and I sat on the examination table trying not to crinkle the neatly placed paper covering—after all, I didn't plan on being there long. The doctor walked in and sat down, which caused his pants' legs to rise, revealing colorful, striped socks and mismatched Converse shoes.

He asked, "What is going on today?"

For a minute, I did not answer because I was too busy chuckling to myself at the thought of being examined by Dr. Seuss.

"My right leg is swollen, and I think I may have a blood clot."

Dr. Seuss proceeded with a physical examination and measured both of my legs. It was clear that one leg was larger than the other, and he ordered an ultrasound. As I made my way to the ultrasound room with the technician, we began chatting about our careers, law school, and our families. I lay down on the examination table in the dark ultrasound room and stared at the posters of kittens and rainbows that had been taped on the ceiling. The lines were faded, but clearly the staff thought they were adequate enough to counterbalance the dismal, gray walls and lack of color.

The test was moving along well, and I continued to chat with the technician until she reached the right side of my pelvis. She examined the area for nearly twenty minutes. This was my first inclination that she had found something out of the ordinary. Her sudden silence was telling, and I asked her what she had found. She looked down at me and explained that she would not be able to answer my question. I understood what this meant, legally at least. It would be a liability for her to discuss this information with me, for her to tell me the truth: that located in my right pelvis she had found—as it would later be described in the medical record by one radiologist—a "massive" tumor, and that I would have to wait for Dr. Seuss' analysis of the scan.

By the time I returned to the examination room, Dr. Seuss had read the scans and entered the room in a frazzled state. I have to admit I was disappointed with his grammatical and verbal skills as he fumbled to find the right words. He was clearly not living up to the name I'd given him. Or his socks.

"Uh... the ultrasound shows a mass in your pelvis, and that's what is causing the swelling in your right leg."

I waited for him to continue, and when he didn't, I asked, "And is that bad?"

"Uh, yeah!" he said with a disturbing amount of distress in his voice. It was clear we were not in Whoville anymore.

"Well, can you elaborate, please?" I asked him nervously and with impatience.

He explained to me that the large mass on the right side of my pelvis was solid, which ruled out the possibility that it could be an ovarian cyst. He went on to explain that he would be referring me to a specialist in gynecological cancers immediately, to undergo a biopsy of the mass to confirm his initial diagnosis: ovarian cancer.

It is at that point that the day blurs for me. Like stop-motion photography, the rest of that day, and indeed, much of the following months is a blur, while other parts remain painfully clear in my memory. For example, I remember how cold it was in the ultrasound room and the exact shade of my mother's lipstick. But I don't remember when my father arrived. I remember him there, his silent presence filling the room as he did an Internet search on his phone, trying to keep up with the information we were being given. I remember he had to leave to go take care of the horses before it got dark, but I don't remember what he said when he left. I have no idea how my mind choose what to retain and what it chose to let slip away, and those blurred moments will probably always bother me. But there was so long that I thought I wouldn't need to remember anything, that I wouldn't live long enough to even consider any of this a memory, that I'm glad for even the gaps.

✦

One of the most difficult things I have ever had to do was to make that first telephone call, to try and explain to my fiancé, Harrison, that the doctor had found a tumor, and he thought it was cancerous. This was a phone call that I knew was going to change not only my life but also Harrison's as well. In an almost serene way, the moments I took to wait to make that first call were moments I cherished. If I could have waited an eternity to make that call, I would have.

Harrison was working as a financial analyst at the time and had to spend a portion of the holidays in Connecticut. Typically, whenever we had holiday vacations, I would go to my parents' ranch in Nevada earlier than him in order to spend a little extra time with my family, and he would later join me. However, because of his job, he had to hear my news while working across the country. He would be thousands of miles away, in shock and with no idea what to do or say, and I felt guilty. I can still feel that sharp twist in my stomach, as if I were choosing to change his life irrevocably.

I couldn't bring myself to call for the first couple of minutes because I imagined him happily sitting on the couch after a hectic day of work. He'd be playing video games or reading one of the ridiculous novels he collected about magicians and magic spells. I wanted nothing more than to give Harrison a few more moments to remain in that mystical world. But my mother and the doctor had given me privacy just for this purpose, so I gathered my courage and collected all my strength. I dialed his phone number.

As the phone rang, I found myself hoping he wouldn't answer. It was just my luck that the one time I was hoping to get Harrison's voicemail, he just happened to see my call (I assure you, this would never have happened if I were calling about dinner reservations, bills, or a flat tire). My strength did not last long; I began to cry as soon as I heard his voice.

Between my sobbing and Harrison frantically asking what was wrong, I apologized profusely. For the first couple of minutes, all I could say was, "I'm sorry, Harrison, I am so sorry." It was easier to worry about him in those first hours.

Finally, when I was able to get out the rest of what I had to say, I said, "They've found a tumor, and the doctor says it's cancer."

Harrison was shocked and began firing off questions, but I didn't have enough answers yet. When my mother came back into the room, I gave her the phone to explain to Harrison everything we knew about what was happening. She sounded calm and reassuring, as she stepped into the hall, his voice, tinny in the phone's inadequate speaker, fading as the door closed behind her and I was left alone.

By the time she came back in, the color bright in her cheeks, her mouth in a tight, forced smile, I had stopped crying. She told me Harrison was doing OK and that we were going to keep him updated. I could only nod. I didn't ask what she'd told him to calm him down, but I wished someone would tell me the same thing.

At that point, we were at the end of the appointment, and a nurse entered the room with a packet. She opened up the packet and explained to us that in these types of situations, when there is such a serious diagnosis, it is common for patients to Google everything they can find about their condition. She informed us that this was the worst thing we could do in terms of forming our strategy and planning together. She recommended that I not search the Internet or do any research on my own until I knew more about my situation in its entirety. We thanked her, and I took the packet of information and walked with my mother out into the cold night air.

It was now dark out, nearly nine o'clock, and the stars shined brightly. It was frigid, and a snowstorm from the recent week had left snow banks along the sides of the roads and parking lot. The ice had melted, and sheets of black ice glistened across the roadways, which were empty at this time of night.

My mother and I climbed into the car. I can't tell you exactly what we said to one another in those initial moments. It's more of the blur. I do remember her anxiety at calling my sister and giving her the news. It was one thing to take the phone from me, to save me from my own hysteria. It was quite another to call her youngest daughter. She'd had time to think about this call and really didn't know what to say.

My mom was always the communicator in the family. Dad took care of the logistics of the household—making sure the checkbook balanced and the horses had enough feed—but mom was the emotional heart. Someone needed to be grounded? My mom would tell us how long. Someone got straight As? My mom was the one to pin the report card on the fridge with flourish. So there was no discussion of who was going to call Alyce.

Earlier in the day, Alyce had called my mom's cell phone to casually check on the outcome of my appointment, but there had been no answer. She had called again an hour later. Nothing. Phone call after phone call went unanswered, and Alyce's dread rose with each passing hour. By midday, she had been desperate for information. She had called our father, only to discover he had already left work at the business he owned in order to be by my side. By the time the barrage of tests were over, we barely made it to the car, completely numb to the world and shaken to our cores.

Alyce was frantic at home, fearing the worst. Finally, my mom called. When she heard Alyce say, "Hello?" my mom could not respond, and I could hear Alyce yelling into the phone. She asked my mother to tell her what had happened, the panic escalating in her voice.

My mother choked up as she managed to explain to Alyce that they had found a tumor, and that I would be seeing a specialist in Reno to undergo tests to confirm that it was malignant. I could hear my sister yelling, "What is going on?" She couldn't understand a word my mother was saying, and her incessant questioning only induced an increasingly dramatic response from my mother. To regain some control over the situation, I grabbed the phone from my mother's hand and yelled the most efficient statement I could: "I'm not dead!"

✦

Within a week after that initial cancer diagnosis, my mom and I met with the gynecological cancer specialist in Reno, Nevada, Dr. Lim, who was confident that it was not ovarian cancer but Hodgkin lymphoma. We went through a variety of possible outcomes, ranging from the best case to the worst. I was scheduled for a biopsy immediately at Saint Mary's Regional

Medical Center in Reno. But it was the thick of the holiday season, and the weeks surrounding Christmas were filled with holiday parties and chaotic family schedules. Scheduling the biopsy was no easy feat as most of the hospital staff, including oncologists and radiologists, were away on vacation. My cancer was not.

Dr. Lim scheduled a biopsy of the mass in my pelvis for a week later, and the preliminary report suggested it was highly suspicious of Hodgkin lymphoma. A simple phone call, that my mom answered. My case files were sent to University of California, San Francisco, for a second opinion.

The week between seeing Dr. Lim and getting the second opinion were spent resting with my leg elevated, as part of some pseudo-medical technique I had developed spontaneously to decrease the swelling. It had been a couple of days since I had been diagnosed, and at this point I was not able to walk due to the size of the tumor in my right hip. It had grown so large that blood was unable to flow back and forth from my leg to the rest of my body.

On January 9, 2012, I was watching the Lifetime television channel, engrossed in a typically saccharine Lifetime movie. The plots of these movies always seemed the same: a woman with a semi-professional job falls in love with a high-powered career man, such as a banker, doctor, or lawyer, who is not invested in the relationship. Somehow the heroine will also have found herself in a devious scandal that could ruin her job and friendships. However, with her wits and common sense, she will find a way to get justice for herself and all the other women who have been slighted by similarly uninvolved and uncaring men. I love these movies.

As I was finishing the movie, my mother ran out of the office and into the living room like a bat out of hell, with more enthusiasm than I could ever have imagined one person could convey. She was crying, but not out of sadness or devastation—out of sheer happiness. Lost in my Lifetime film, I was completely oblivious to what had been going on around me and looked at her, confused. Through her happy tears, she exclaimed, "It's Hodgkin's lymphoma! It's Hodgkin's lymphoma! It is HODGKIN'S!"

I was surprised by her excitement. It was like watching a car accident, all the cars demolished and piled up on the side of the road. It's horrifying, but then, amid all the chaos, out of the corner of your eye you catch a glimpse of the family standing beside the wreckage, and you think, "Thank God they survived." My mother was so thrilled because I had the "right kind" of cancer.

✦

The oncology and hematology practice in Reno, Nevada, was located in an antiquated medical building with dilapidated floors and defective elevators. A sign hanging on the elevator door read, "Under Repair." I laughed at the sign as I made my way to the fourth floor, thinking, *Aren't we all?* The lower levels of the building were occupied by various clinics, including an OBGYN practice. As I went through my treatment, I took many elevator rides with pregnant women.

It did not seem strange in the beginning, but once cancer treatment began to take hold, I noticed a peculiar paradox. Here we would be, two young women standing in an elevator, both preparing for two of the most important issues we all must face: life and death. We never spoke—there was always a degree of distance—and the most we ever shared was a polite smile. While she celebrated a budding new life, I stared at my potential mortality.

The waiting room was small, the chairs were old, and the walls were discolored and brown. I waited with my mother below a huge quote painted on the wall, proclaiming, "While cancer can take most things in your life, it cannot quench the spirit!" I winced every time I read that quote and thought it was insulting that they'd had the audacity to paint it on the wall. I couldn't help but think how many people had passed away who had once sat in this very room, staring at that phrase while waiting to receive chemotherapy treatment—people who thought, *Screw this sign.*

I was called into the back office, and my mom watched as the nurse took my weight. I weighed 119 pounds, as expected. We followed the same nurse into a dreary, outdated walk-in closet. I sat on the examination table and my mom took the chair in the corner behind the door, and we waited for the doctor. I was curious to meet my new oncologist, Dr. Reese, but I was not quite prepared for what would happen next.

The door swung open and nearly slammed my mother in the nose. In walked a young Indian man in his early thirties.

He sat down without introduction or preamble, looked me straight in the face, and said, "Your biopsy results came back, and I am sorry, but it is cancer. Your PET scan results have also shown that the cancer has spread outside of the pelvic region and has metastasized to the liver. I am sorry, but it is stage IV."

I had been prepared for Dr. Reese to confirm that I had cancer. But stage IV? He went on to tell me that without immediate treatment, this cancer would kill me within thirty days. I remember that clearly. But it didn't quite click at the time.

"Well, I would like to have surgery so you can remove the cancer," I said. "However, we need to do it fast because I have to be back in Connecticut for law school on January 16. We are beginning our spring semester, and I have to recover by then."

Dr. Reese said nothing for a moment, and then in a soft voice he said, "Sarah, surgery is not an option. You have cancer throughout your entire lymphatic system."

I was growing frustrated. "You can treat this, right?"

"Yes, Sarah. You are going to need to start chemotherapy right away. The standard regimen for your type of cancer is called ABVD, a combination chemotherapy made up of the chemotherapies Adriamycin, Bleomycin, Vinblastine, and Dacarbazine. The treatment will take six months."

I almost fell off the examination table, "Six months? What do you mean 'six months?' I have law school! I live in Connecticut!"

The room had fallen silent before Dr. Reese responded. "Sarah, I am sorry, but you will not be able to return to law school."

I tried desperately to choke back my fear, rage, and tears. In that one moment, I lost everything. In one unforeseen swipe, my life was changed forever. It became unrecognizable. But more than that, it wasn't even anything I could imagine. I had cancer, but there weren't going to be any pink ribbons or races for the cure for me. Not in thirty days.

My mother broke the silence. "Should I take her to Stanford? We can leave today."

Dr. Reese replied, "No, no, I have already spoken to Stanford, and they said there is no need for you to go there because they would prescribe the same treatment." Dr. Reese appeared peeved when he answered the question, as if he were against losing me as a patient to Stanford.

When I finally gathered myself together, I calmly asked the only question I could think of: "Am I going to lose my hair?" I pulled at the long, brown strands that fell past my shoulders.

"Yes. Most patients choose not to cut their hair before it begins to fall out—but some shave their heads. They feel it is less traumatic."

I saw my reflection in the glass of a picture frame tried to imagine myself bald. I thought, *Less traumatic? What is this man thinking?* Then I imagined myself standing in the shower or brushing my hair, pulling clumps from my scalp and holding the limp strands between my fingers. It broke my heart, but hell if I was going to let the beautiful hair that I had spent years growing and nurturing go to waste. I decided I would get a pixie cut and donate my hair to Locks of Love, a foundation that makes wigs for cancer patients. I could do that even if I only had thirty days.

Dr. Reese interrupted my thought process. "Sarah, you are going to need to get a PowerPort placed in your chest within the next few days. The PowerPort will be used to administer your chemotherapy treatments, and, in case of emergency, it enables us to inject large quantities of medication quickly and safely into your system, should this at any point become necessary. Additionally, the port also serves to protect your body's ventricular system from the harsh properties of the chemotherapy treatment. However, first thing Monday morning, you are scheduled to come in for a bone marrow biopsy, which I will perform here in the office to determine whether or not your bone marrow indicates that the cancer has metastasized to your bones."

By this point, I was so exhausted and worn down that I was no longer interested in questioning what he was telling me, and I quietly agreed.

✦

That weekend after learning I had stage IV cancer, we had a family party. I have a large family, with thirteen aunts and uncles and more cousins than I could possibly count. For them, I wore a party hat.

Hodgkin lymphoma is typically highly responsive, with a 90–95 percent cure rate. Even at stage IV, it was good news. That thirty days had only been if I didn't get treatment, which seemed ludicrous to me.

I didn't quite know how to react to any of it. It was strange to have received a stage IV cancer diagnosis and yet be told that I should be grateful and that I was blessed. Clearly, this had been the type of cancer that we had all been praying for, as twisted as that may sound.

✦

My mother and I returned to the office a few days later for the bone marrow biopsy. Dr. Reese, accompanied by a nurse practitioner, told me, "Do not worry, Sarah. I do this all of the time. It will feel like a bee sting."

This analogy did not put me at ease. I wanted a bit more clarification. "Well, Dr. Reese I have never been stung by a bee, so I don't know how that is going to feel. Have you ever been stung by a bee?"

"Well, no," he admitted, "I haven't, Sarah."

"Then how do you know it feels like a bee sting? What if it's horrible? Can you give me another reference?"

Dr. Reese looked at me impatiently, so I relented and did as he instructed and lay face down on the examination table. I looked over at the nurse and saw the largest needle I had ever seen in my life.

"Good lord! Is that what you're going to use? *That* feels like a bee sting?"

I gripped the examination table harder and squeezed my eyes shut as the nurse first numbed the area and then attempted to insert the needle into my hip bone. I screamed out in pain. The needle could not penetrate the hard bone and bent in half.

"We are going to try again," Dr. Reese said, attempting to sound authoritative.

I looked at the nurse and then at Dr. Reese. I started to doubt this man's judgment. "Are you sure you know what you're doing? Are you sure you're going to get it this time?"

Dr. Reese was clearly flustered. "Yes, but you need to stop yelling; you are scaring the other patients."

I looked up at Dr. Reese and responded firmly, "They *should* be scared."

I felt another bolt of searing pain, shrieked out once again, and for a second time the needle would not penetrate the bone. Before I could object to continuing this painful procedure, an older doctor burst through the door. It was Dr. Shefield, Dr. Reese's superior, one of the two founding oncologists of the practice.

"What's going on in here?" she asked with an irritated tone.

"We cannot get the needle to go into the bone," Dr. Reese replied.

Dr. Shefield's jaw tightened angrily, "Well, stop trying! Why are you doing this here? She needs to get it done at the hospital as an outpatient procedure!" With that, Dr. Shefield turned on her heel and left and indignantly shut the door behind her.

I looked at Dr. Reese and the nurse. "You mean that was all for nothing?"

Not in the least bit concerned, Dr. Reese calmly began to explain: "We cannot get the needle to go into your hip bone, and we will have to schedule an outpatient procedure. We will have it scheduled right before your port placement in the morning."

I left the appointment bruised, sore, and with diminished confidence in my oncologist. I was angry that he had put me through that procedure in the office rather than sending me to the hospital in the first place. That morning was the first time I began to question whether Dr. Reese and I were a good match.

✦

Before I was to go for round two of the biopsy and port placement, I needed to have three tests done. These three tests—the echocardiogram, pulmonary function, and ultrasound tests—were used to measure the function of my heart, my lungs, and my ventricular systems, the main organ systems of my body.

The echocardiogram was not terribly dull, but it was awkward at first. A young male technician was the one to adhere the cold strips to my chest and abdomen and then hook me up as if he were about to jumpstart his car. It took a good ten minutes to get past the intimacy of it, but then the whole thing was rather pleasant. We talked about a myriad of things, ranging from education, to politics, to our careers, to spouses (and future spouses). I didn't know it then, but this would be one of the last times a young man treated me like an average twenty-something-year-old female and…wait for it…did not want to engage in some psychology 101 experiment and spend the hour discussing my cancer.

The pulmonary function test was my least favorite. I've never had particularly strong lungs, and I felt like a failed astronaut inside the glass cylinder, losing oxygen and hyperventilating. On the walls of the pulmonary suite were those terrible motivational posters, usually with a puppy or kitten, that said, "Just Breathe." *Forget you! Just breathe? I am about to give myself a brain aneurysm if I have to give it another go.* It quickly went from the little engine that could—I think I can, I think I can—to the little engine that could not.

The ultrasound was done by a woman, and because the pelvic region was the initial site of metastasis, this would become the longest gynecological exploration, not just appointment, on record (at least it felt that way to me). It was obvious what she saw on the screen was bad, and she distracted me (and maybe herself) with explaining how the ultrasound worked. She likened it to astronomy. The Doppler effect is at the crux of it all, and I found it interesting enough to keep the atmosphere as light as possible during the probings.

✦

The day of the PowerPort placement, my mother and I left the house early and drove to Saint Mary's in Reno. The nurse explained to me that I would have the bone marrow biopsy first, and then they would wheel me down the hall to radiology, where they would place my new PowerPort. It all sounded like a reasonable plan in the beginning.

The surgeon's assistant took me into the first room for the bone marrow biopsy. Glancing at the medical team, I asked their names and who was going to do what, when, where, and how. I always feel better when I know what to expect. And with stage IV cancer, there wasn't much of that, so I grasped it wherever and whenever I could.

The team explained who they each were, that they were going to sedate me, and that at the most I would feel a slight pressure as the machine, guided by one of the team members, penetrated my hip bone. I hoped the needle on the machine was stronger than the one at Dr. Reese's office.

They told me they were going to use conscious sedation, and they said it like it was a good thing. But I looked at the team member administering the medication and explained that I have a very high tolerance for anesthesia and would need a considerable amount of medication to get through the two procedures. I'd been through it the year before, when I'd sliced into my hand trying to get fancy cutting an avocado. I'd had to have surgery to reconnect severed nerves and woken halfway through. It was horrifying, and I didn't want to go through it again.

I told the anesthesiologist it was imperative that he watch me for signs I was coming out of the anesthesia because I would wake up during the procedure if he didn't administer enough medication. He told me not to worry, and I began to feel lethargic and sleepy and briefly nodded off. However, as sure as sunrise, I woke up and looked straight into the eyes of the anesthesiologist. I felt a deep pressure pierce my hip bone, and I reached out for his hand, in shock from the pain. I gritted my teeth and tried to hold perfectly still, gripping his hand, knowing it was too late to stop the procedure.

This time the needle was able to penetrate the bone and, while excruciating, the marrow aspiration was successful. It hadn't taken more than a few minutes, but it felt like hours.

Once the biopsy was complete, the medical team rolled me over onto my back and prepared me for the PowerPort placement in the upper right of my chest. They would be inserting the port, which was about the size of a silver dollar, with a tube that was threaded through the central venous line. The anesthesiologist administered more medication and I slipped into unconsciousness before the orderly wheeled me into the second room to start the procedure.

As the radiologist placing the port made the first incision into my chest, I awoke again. I began to breathe quickly and frantically, and I heard a nurse call out, "She's awake; we have to stop the procedure!" I could not see the radiologist's face because it was shielded by a blue sheet that served as a barrier between the two of us. The radiologist stopped immediately.

"No," I managed to mutter. "No, I'm starting chemotherapy tomorrow morning. You have to finish the procedure now."

The radiologist said, "All right, but you have to stop moving. Please be completely still and try not to tense your muscles, or else I won't be able to place the port."

A nurse came to my side, and I reached out and took her hand. The radiologist continued. As the scalpel cut through each of the ligaments and muscles, I squeezed the nurse's hand tighter and focused on keeping my body still. My muscles were releasing like spring-loaded levers. As I turned my head to the left, tears streaming down my face, I caught a glimpse of the anesthesiologist from the first procedure walking past the room. We locked eyes, and he stopped; we stared at each other for what felt like hours. He winced as he stood on the other side of the glass. Even under the circumstances, I could see how terrible he felt having not given me enough anesthesia in the prior procedure, and then witnessing the agony of the second.

Once the port was placed, I waited for the radiologist and his team to leave the room before I broke down and began to sob uncontrollably right there on the table. The radiologist came quickly back into the room. "What's wrong?" he said with a strong sense of urgency and concern. "You fell asleep for most of the procedure."

I looked up at him and, through my tears, I managed to reply, "No, I didn't. I was awake the whole time."

The radiologist's disposition changed instantly. It became soft, comforting, and personal. He leaned across the table in an almost fatherly way and gently said, "It's over now. Why are you so upset? Is it your hair?"

I looked up at him disbelievingly. "No. I have cancer, and I'm only twenty-four years old."

He paused and seemed to grapple with something before speaking. "You know, Sarah, my daughter has just completed cancer treatment for stage IV non-Hodgkin lymphoma. She is just a bit younger than you, and I remember when she lost her hair, she cut it short like yours, and then we bought her a wig at Tiffany's Tresses. She hated her short hair, but she looked beautiful. My daughter was in the hospital for twelve straight weeks receiving chemotherapy this past spring. She was scared, and I was terrified. I'm so happy to tell you that she is in remission and will begin school at the University of Nevada, Reno, this fall. I know you're scared, but you're going to be just fine. You will beat this."

As he was telling me the story, I was thinking WTF? Did he not get what I'd been through? Did he not understand the trauma of waking during a procedure like that? But just after he left the room, a nurse came in and was in disbelief that he had told me such a personal story, especially one that was such a recent wound for him. In that moment, I realized he was trying to connect with me. His touchstone for the horror of what I was facing was not the same as mine. He understood my trauma because his daughter had gone through it. But anesthesia was his job. My horrific experience was just part of the job. A horrible part, but not anything he hadn't seen before. Hair loss, however: that he had only known through his daughter. And it had been what made her cancer real, so he was sharing that with me to let me know he understood just how real it was about to get.

The radiologist surprised me. He was the first person ever to tell me a personal cancer story, and it gave me courage and comfort to know that his daughter had gone through a similar situation and was now in remission. I would in later months remind myself often of the radiologist and his daughter, envisioning her bright, healthy, and enjoying her time at the university. It was these particular moments that I would come to hold onto, and it was here that I found hope when it was all but absent.

# CHAPTER TWO

# ROOTS

*I come from a proud line of women who relentlessly pursued their passions.*

✦

Most of my life I spent looking forward. I'd achieve one goal and immediately move onto the next. If one were easy to accomplish, the next one would be harder. Because of that, my resume looks more akin to that of a fifty year old than someone half that age. But it wasn't until I was diagnosed with cancer that I started to really look at who I was and how I wanted to live. There always seemed time for that later. But while cancer introduces a whole flock of words into one's vocabulary, "later" isn't one of them.

After I had the port placed, my cancer became very real to me. Suddenly there was this physical reminder, this intrusion on my body, this cheery purple plastic reminder of death that I couldn't ignore. I blame the port for making me so nostalgic and introspective in those beginning days of treatment. I needed to analyze who I had been so I could figure out who I needed to become to survive.

My family lived on a small ranch in a rural town in Nevada. With mud on my boots and dust in my hair, I spent my days racing through sagebrush with my first playmate, a gray and white dusted quarter horse named Babe.

By the time I was six years old, my younger sister and I qualified for the first time to compete in the rodeo. Every week we traded our Catholic school uniforms for Ariat boots and jeans and kicked the dirt off our heels as we sat on the sidewalk. We watched our classmates pile into various minivans and SUVs while we waited for the horse trailer that carried each of our horses to practice. The training was difficult and time-consuming. For the next few years, I traveled with my mother and sister in an incessant cycle on the state and national rodeo circuits, competing, training, refining, and perfecting my riding technique.

The training was strenuous and often competition was painful; to compete at the level that my sister and I did required sacrifice and dedication. Training took up the majority of our time, leaving little room for interests elsewhere. I definitely learned how to focus.

One of the difficult lessons that I learned through training and competition is that there are good days and there are bad days. There were days where I was on fire, and swept through the wins. However, there were also days where I lost no matter how hard I tried. I made a mistake or someone on my team was off or sometimes my horse and I would simply be out of sync.

Regardless of whether I won or lost, it was challenging because I had to do so with grace, humility, and good sportsmanship. It was easy to have good spirits on the days when the wins seemed to be stacking up, but it was in the days of loss where my true colors shown. Learning to be not only a good winner, but also a good loser has played a fundamental part in the development of my character today. It may seem simple enough, but in practice it was far more difficult than it appeared.

The rewards, lessons learned, and characteristics I developed justified my years of rough training and difficult losses. However, as invested as I had become in the rodeo, I dreamed of greater achievements, influential writers, opera composers, and beautiful cities.

At the age of twelve I found myself saddling up my horse with my competition number in one hand and an opera score in the other, tapping out the rhythm of the masterpieces of Puccini and Verdi, waiting to be called on deck for my run. It'd been awhile since I lost, and racing had become second nature. Only when my name was called over the loudspeaker, did I hand off my sheet music to my nearby trainer. I approached the gate and positioned my heels in my stirrups. In a split second, I lunged into a low, supported, aerodynamic position as my horse approached the first turn. But my mind was filled with words and music. It wouldn't be long before I traded passions.

By the time I was sixteen, I was ready for college, where I could explore multiple avenues at once. Five years later, I had a triple bachelor's degree (economics, political science, and sociology). I had just begun my law school when I got my cancer diagnosis. That changed everything—except my drive.

✦

I come from a proud line of women who relentlessly pursued their passions. During the long rodeo weekends, while other kids were outside roping each other's heels and spurs, I sat in the bleachers reading my mom's old university textbooks and reports she wrote on suffrage. I also became absorbed in the case files she had saved from her career as a detective.

My mother, Sue Coffey, was the first woman to be assigned to the patrol division in Carson City, Nevada, and specialized in child sexual abuse at the Carson City Sheriff's Office. During her career, she was notorious for accepting the most difficult cases and still holding the highest confession rate in her department—all while raising three young children with her husband, a sergeant in that same office. Her work established two legislative statutes in Nevada, both reactions to notorious criminal cases involving child neglect and sexual abuse. Her dedication was recognized by the *Wall Street Journal*, *Good Morning America*, and most recently was mentioned on a popular television show on reconstructive surgery: *Dr. 90210* (as a detective, she had saved the life of a little girl who had been attacked by her family's pet ferret)

Relentlessly upholding her principles, my mother pursued each case with unparalleled commitment and perseverance, dedicating those years of her life to the victims and their families.

As I watched my mother over the years, proud of her achievements and listened to her stories of her own mother, I realized it was my grand-mother who had been at the forefront of shaping my mother's convictions and principles.

Mary Coffey, my grandmother, had found the strength to leave her destructive marriage and went on to support her seven children on a secretary's salary. She never remarried. Instead, she became a key figure in the fight for pay equity in the state of Nevada. She was even honored for her pursuit of women's equality at a reception held by President Jimmy Carter at the White House.

Tucked away in my family home on the ranch in Nevada, I spent hours combing through pictures of my grandmother at conventions and women's rights rallies. It wasn't until 2013, when I read the works of Sandra Day O'Connor, that I learned my grandmother's connection to the Supreme Court Justice was more than just traveling in the same women's rights circles. They fought side by side. I was proud to read that Justice O'Connor listed my grandmother as one of her heroes.

One of my proudest moments was standing by my grandmother's side when she was eighty-nine at a ceremony held in her honor by Harry Reid and the Nevada democrats. I listened to several political figures pay tribute to her and discuss how my grandmother motivated them to take action for the rights of women.

These days if I want to look at those pictures, I head to the archives at the University of Nevada, Reno, where her life's work as an activist are available for university and public research. I'm obviously not alone in thinking of her as a truly great woman.

I always knew I had big shoes to fill. When I found out I might not have as much time to fill them as I had always assumed, I had to completely re-analyze what I wanted in the world and how I could best bring it about. But first, I had to put all my focus on surviving. Something I had always pretty much accomplished without effort was now going to take everything I had ever learned, everything I ever was. I needed to understand myself just to know what skills I brought to the table. If I were going to bet on me, I couldn't bluff. Not with this much on the line.

# CHAPTER THREE

# THE ACTIVE PATIENT

*Silence.*
*Unnecessary and unfair. One of cancer's most malicious and cunning killers.*

✦

At the beginning of my cancer treatment, I was like many patients in that I gave substantial discretion and authority to my first team of oncologists in Reno, Nevada, and did not question their decisions regarding my treatment. It stayed this way through the biopsy and chemotherapy, through recurrence of my cancer and more chemotherapy, until I assumed the role of an active patient. I finally learned that I was my strongest advocate and needed to be included on decisions made, not only about my health, but medical decisions that would ultimately, had I not challenged them, cost me my life.

Even after being unrelenting in my legal career, having competed on the rodeo circuit, and traveling internationally to sing Opera, I still fell right into passive mode when it came to doctors. But as I was looking back (maybe because it was easier than looking forward), I was thinking a lot about the strong women who had come before me. I tried to imagine my grandmother or even my mother facing a death sentence. I thought of my mom taking on a child abuse ring. I thought of my grandmother choosing divorce in a time when women did not do that (especially women with seven children to feed). Then I tried to imagine either of them sitting in a doctor's office, vulnerable in a paper gown, scared, confused. What would they do if someone told them they were going to die soon? But I couldn't imagine them cowering. I'm pretty sure there would be a lot of questions—and no small amount of profanity if those questions weren't adequately answered.

In 2010, had anyone asked me, I would've told him or her I'd be the same way. I'd be getting second opinions and interrogating anyone who wanted to do anything with my body. I'd be researching and reading case histories and stalking scientists.

But come 2011, with a stage IV diagnosis, I came very close to folding. The diagnosis knocked me on my heels. The aggressive timeline for my treatment flummoxed the student in me. And feeling so far out of my element made it easy for me to slip into a passive role I had never been in before. I didn't even know I had that in me.

Let me be clear here, though: questioning one's doctors and insisting on being included in medical decisions is *not* the same as ignoring one's physician. On the contrary, the active patient actively searches out specialists and maintains open lines of communication. The patient is able to speak to, clarify, and consult with physicians who are experts in their fields. The goal is for the patient and the physicians to work together to become a single interdependent team.

Active patients also interact with support systems such as web communities, nurses, and case managers. No stone is left unturned when it comes to the search for care. While the physicians and the patient are the brain and heart of the team, they are nourished by information, ideas, and support from an extensive network of sources.

Interactive web communities allow the patient to post messages and receive replies from patients all over the world who are experiencing similar situations. This helps the patients remember they are not alone (because they aren't).

Local support groups allow people with similar ailments to meet in person and discuss their issues with others who have gone through the same things.

Nurses and case managers make up the backbone of the team. They often spend more time with patients than the doctors do and become allies in ways the doctors' needed objectivity doesn't allow. They can be advocates and confidantes. Nurses and cases managers are there to be a comfort to the patient as well as provide guidance on the roadmap of treatment.

Friends, family, and caregivers can provide crucial support, and it is tempting to let one or all of them take the central role of advocate. But the active patient knows how to be his or her own medical advocate.

In the beginning, I let my mom drive me to appointments and take care of my prescriptions. She kept my schedule and even made sure I ate. It was comforting. It was easy. But the more I let her take care of me, the more passive I became. The more passive I became, the more mistakes were made. I eventually had to take center stage in my own treatment. That doesn't mean I didn't ever have my mom drive me home after chemo or let my sister run to the pharmacy. And I never turned down anyone who wanted to bring me food. The difference was that I asked for or accepted their help. I switched from just experiencing their help to being the gatekeeper of that help. People were no longer doing things *to* me, they were doing things *for* me.

Here are some basic things active patients do to assist in their own health care. For example, know how to get to your doctor's office. If you drive yourself, give yourself plenty of time to arrive and park, so you're not frazzled for your appointment causing extra anxiety by being late or not being able to find parking. Even if you have someone drive you, be sure that you know the way. There's nothing wrong with asking for and accepting help, just don't let that be a reason to not know the way. Understand everything, but it's fine to not do everything.

Write down all of the questions you have for doctors and support staff in advance. This way you will not forget anything vital you need to ask your doctor, nurse, or case manager. Don't know what questions to ask? Be an active patient by asking about your treatment. How can you best prepare for treatment? How long will it take? Can you go to and from treatment alone or do you need someone to drive you? Can you have a loved one or caregiver present during treatment? What are the side effects of the treatment? After treatment, what should you watch for and what symptoms should make you call the doctor?

Additionally, write down anything you may want to tell your doctor, such as new pain or discomfort or that you're switching to a different pharmacy. Write it down before your appointment so that you can focus on new information being given rather than remembering everything you meant to ask. Keep a list between appointments and bring that list with you when you see the doctor.

Make sure to keep a folder or binder of all of your health information and bring this folder to each oncology appointment, adding to it as your treatment progresses. This way you will always have any medical information at hand when you need it.

Keep a list of all of your prescription medications and dosages with you in your medical folder. Also, write down how often you take the medication and what time of day you take it. On the same sheet of paper, write down which doctor is prescribing which medication as well as which pharmacy or pharmacist is filling it. If possible, get all of your medications from one pharmacy. This will help you build a relationship with your pharmacist as well as make it easy for your oncologist to know where to call to dispense refills or help you with any errors. Your pharmacist is also an integral part of your medical team and can help catch medication interactions and allergies.

While talking to the doctor or health team, if you don't understand a question or answer, ask them to rephrase it for you. Don't sit back and let it slip past you without taking the time to understand it. If you need to ask more, take your full appointment time to ask questions. If you are stressed out or worried, let your doctor or nurse know what your worries are and make sure they are addressed. Your doctor's office should have numerous resources available to you. But they don't always know which ones you need unless you speak up.

Before you leave the office, know what the next steps are for your care, whether it be a specific treatment, medication, or follow-up visit. One way to ensure you never miss this kind of information is to take notes during your doctor's appointments or ask a loved one or caregiver to do it for you.

Record everything—visits with doctors, case workers, and their medical teams. It will help you keep organized and will allow you to refer back to important medical information should the occasion arise. Do not trust your memory alone. Nothing overwhelms your available bandwidth like the complexity of cancer.

✦

Most people don't know the exact moment during their life that they made a choice to become the exception or the rule. In my extreme case, it was making that choice that ultimately dictated whether I would live or die.

Right now being an active patient is the exception. Our medical system is predicated on the medical staff being the center of treatment. They make the decisions, chart a course of action, and execute it, often without getting more than a signature from the patient. I am ready for change.

One of the greatest minds that I have ever met and had the privilege of knowing in my life, stayed passive, and it killed her. Claire will forever be one of the greatest inspirations and reasons for why I have chosen to dedicate my life to the work that I do.

This brilliant woman, this life force, this beacon of an individual, who I could only hope to one day aspire to even being just glimmer of, knew which moment in her life, what second determined whether she would live or die. Weak from chemotherapy and cancer treatment, Claire chose not to speak. She had been assigned a course of treatment that she knew didn't make sense. It was untested and counter-intuitive. But she was so tired and so deferential to her doctors (in ways she was with no one else in her life) that she chose to mention her quite valid concerns. She remained silent. It was just a second, just a brief single moment in time. However, in the end that was the only one that truly mattered. She went ahead with a treatment she didn't trust.

I watched her waste away and gradually try to come to terms with the decision that was made at the moment that cost her life.

She died replaying that moment in her mind, over and over, changing all the variables like an econometric regression analysis, seeing if the results were different, but in the end they were all the same.

Silence.

Death.

Unnecessary and unfair. Silence is one of cancer's most malicious and cunning killers. Do not remain silent. In silence, you may lose the only moment that matters, the one when you should have spoken.

I thought of her during my treatment—one more strong, exemplary woman to add to my roster of heroes. I was so scared of not learning from her mistake and thereby not honoring her life that I knew the moment my speaking saved me.

She showed me how to save myself, and every time I took the reins and saved myself I thought of her. I had an autologous bone marrow transplant and because my cancer had not spread to my bone marrow nor spread to my brain I was able to use my own stem cells for my own transplant. Therefore, I did not require a donor. I saved myself.

I saved myself when I reached the point when I was reconciling my own death alone in a dark hospital room.

I saved myself when I woke up and realized that I had not died and was full of dread, anger, and frustration. This because I did not want to have to go through what it would be like to learn to live again. This would mean I would have to learn to save myself all over again.

I saved myself when I argued with a doctor who wanted to base my treatment on his incorrect memory and refused to check my file to see if he were right. When it really came down to the boots hitting the pavement, I saved myself. But every time, I thought of my friend.

# CHAPTER FOUR

# THEORY TO PRACTICE

*Treatment often comes with unexpected turns, failures, and triumphs. It helps to take it week by week, and as Dr. Ginna Laport, professor of medicine at Stanford University Medical Center would say, "Don't borrow sorrow from tomorrow."*

✦

Any cancer diagnosis is overwhelming and life changing. Oftentimes, we patients find ourselves unable to process mentally the entire gambit of information, treatment, prognosis, and all the steps we must take. It is common when a patient becomes overwhelmed by the enormity of the diagnosis, that everything becomes too much to bear. "Chunking it" has for me as a patient, been the most effective approach. It is easy to let the mind run with hundreds of possible scenarios, but focusing on each individual phase of my treatment enabled me to psychologically break down my situation into "chunks" of manageable pieces. Whenever my mind would start to wander ahead, I'd simply promise myself that I would explore all those what-ifs when I got to whatever stage was worrying me, but for the time being I would stick to the information I needed for this particular stage of my climb. I'd find my footing, move carefully ahead, and just not look down.

Dr. Ginna Laport, from the Stanford University Medical Center, is one of the most phenomenal people that I have been blessed to have in my life. Dr. Laport's approach to the treatment of cancer and the patient's role throughout the cancer treatment was unlike anything I had experienced with any of my prior physicians. I wish I had found her sooner. But it wouldn't be until after an argument with one of my doctors over the size of my tumor that I would realize how fallible medical practitioners could be. While that argument had been devastating at the time, it was finally got my case transferred to Stanford and what ultimately bought me the time I have left.

I was never just part of the cancer assembly line to Dr. Laport. When I wanted to lay in bed and sleep for days and stop exercising from the pain of the Neupogen shots or the fatigue from the chemotherapy or radiation, Dr. Laport said no. When I was depressed in a dark place, where the only thing that I wanted to do was curl up in my bed in my room and never move again, Dr. Laport did not allow my behavior. She told me to get up. She said if I felt like running ten miles, then I should run ten miles. If I felt like walking a mile, then I should walk a mile. But what I could not do was wallow in bed lying around all day, because that was one of the worst things that I could do to my body.

However, following my bone marrow transplant, almost ten months and several rounds of chemo into my treatment, I felt too exhausted, too fatigued, and was too stubborn to get up and even walk down the hall or do the exercises on a stationary bike for even three minutes a day.

My life had fallen apart. I had lost everything, and my future looked nothing like I had planned. I couldn't do the simplest activities that I used to love. I couldn't watch any of my favorite old legal movies or any remotely challenging television shows because it would make me sick to my stomach. I couldn't look at any type of social media, because I would see people just like the old me, young women living beautiful lives, while mine so delicately dangled from a thread.

Dr. Laport was tough as nails. Even when I threw in the towel, had exhausted my caregivers, and terrorized the nursing staff at the Stanford Medical Center, I was no match for Dr. Laport. Now I will admit, in the moment it felt like Dr. Laport's approach was a bit uncompromising. But in the end it really was tough love. Dr. Laport challenged me to get out of bed, to stay in the present moment, not to be a drama queen, and ultimately to stop watching *The Real Housewives of Orange County* because "those women just make mountains out of molehills."

Dr. Laport was the first physician that not only believed I would survive, but believed in my survival even when I didn't believe it myself. When I didn't want to survive, she was the reminder for both me and my family that this wasn't over and that I would go on to live a long, happy life.

She was tough, but she was also my cheerleader, and she taught me one of the most valuable lessons I learned about handling my cancer: "chunking it." Chunking it has, been the most effective approach to managing the overwhelming circumstances surrounding my cancer diagnosis. It was easy to let the mind run with hundreds of possible scenarios, however focusing on each individual part of my treatment enabled me to psychologically break down my situation into "bite-sized" manageable pieces. One chunk at a time. This helped to keep me in the present moment, not focusing on my trying to get back to school or work or my tasks within a six-month or a year range but what I needed to overcome today, tomorrow, this week. What could I do today that would give me the best chance at survival in the long run. Dr. Laport's approach of chunking it had me examine my life as it came to me: in manageable pieces. As she would tell me whenever I started worrying too far ahead, "Don't borrow sorrow from tomorrow."

When I was first diagnosed with cancer, I was inundated with an overwhelming amount of news. Not only was I receiving a large amount of medical information from my medical teams regarding my condition, but I was also given information on support groups, counseling, non-profits, health insurance, and financial assistance.

The medical terms and language alone were overwhelming, not to mention the descriptions of the treatments, medications, side effects, and prognoses. Researching on my own helped me retain a sense of control over the situation and gave me the language I would need for talking with my doctors. I printed out web pages and took extensive notes, just as I had in preparation for law school finals. The familiar ground was strangely comforting.

But I was careful with where I got information.

When I play back the recording of that first urgent care visit, I hear the nurse's soft voice. "I know that you are going to want to go home tonight and Google this information. I know you're scared, and this is a very frightening time. However, the absolute worst thing that you can do at this point is to go online and search for all the possibilities. Sarah, what you will find is a great deal of misinformation and skewed statistics that will do nothing but cause you to worry and panic even more. Now, if you absolutely must go online, make sure that you remain strictly on the .gov (government), .edu (education), or .org (medical and professional) websites, and stay away from the .com websites."

I turned to the Internet anyway as the only source of peace after the barrage of input I had received. But I quickly saw how slippery the slope was for falling into the rabbit hole of outdated, and skewed information, platitudes and miracle cures, and good information that just didn't apply to my situation. Whenever the information started to seem too broad, too suspect or even too emotional, I went back to the .edu and .gov sites and branched out from there. It didn't take long for me to narrow down the useful sites to those about my specific cancer, those ran by groups of people in my same shoes, and those that understood the science behind treatment. Though I am a woman of deep faith, I didn't have time or patience for miracles, especially on sites run by people trying to sell them.

When I switched medical teams, leaving behind Reno and Drs. Reese and Shefield, I asked my new medical team at Stanford where they would recommend I turn for information. They gave me the same answer. They warned me to stay away from .coms and cancer blogs as well. By modifying their advice and sticking to its spirit, I was able to spare myself a great deal of anxiety-provoking information that did not reflect or apply to my diagnosis. The information gleaned from the .gov, .edu, and .org sites provided useful references and contact information that was helpful when I was ready to take on more information and step into the active patient role.

✦

There was a period of time during my cancer treatment where I was still able to attend law school. Strangely, the two—cancer treatment and law school—played off each other. The pressures of studying for my classes prepared me for studying my cancer. Being active in trials helped me eventually become an active patient. My discipline in short-term struggle for long-term goals prepared me for chunking it. But it went the other way too.

When I was in law school, I was president (or "Justice," as we called it) of the legal organization Phi Alpha Delta. I had been a member of the organization for several years as a pre-law student before attending law school. Once I began law school, I became an officer.

One of the tenets of Phi Alpha Delta was the importance of strong professional programs. This was a challenge because there was talk among the local law firms that the law students understood the theory of law just fine. (That is, the law we were taught in our textbooks and in the classrooms was good enough.) However, there was a large learning curve during internships, and this learning curve was costing the law firms time and money in unexpected training costs because what the students had been taught in the classroom was not translating well in real world practice.

We law students were hearing the same thing. The rumor mill was rife with stories of incredibly smart and talented graduates who could not perform a proper handshake or speak in front of room of clients and opposing council. We heard about fellow students who had never had a real job and didn't know how to fill out a timesheet. Career Services at the school had started a series of lectures and seminars to address the simplest of these problems.

This gave me an idea to start a program that I called the Theory to Practice Program. It is one thing to learn the tenets and the details of any theory or philosophy of any type of specific law or application, but it is a completely different ball game to take that theory and actually put it into practice. The real world comes with unexpected events and crises that can blindside a person even after that person thought every possible risk scenario had been considered. It is not enough just to understand the theory. People need to be able to apply what they have learned in the real world and work with what cards they have been dealt. The theories are the tools; people must also know how to use them. One chunk at a time.

With cancer, the theory I embraced was that of being an active patient. I needed to take charge of my life at a time when it felt as if I had no control. I saw it as comparable to rock climbing. In climbing, what's scary is often not how far we have to go but how far from our base we've come. It's the whole reason we're told not to look down. It's not the height; it's the realization that how far we have come is an indicator of how far we could fall. Is the goal worth that risk?

Mine was, in theory. But in practice, it was hard. The more active I became, the easier it was to not look down, but I never completely got over that fear of heights. Instead, I used that fear to explore more theory, finding information a strong rope with which I could pull myself forward.

Chunking it had allowed me to avoid looking down and grapple with one problem at a time, gain one skill at a time. It was the same for the law students.

The Theory to Practice Program soon became not only a resource for learning, but also a sort of matchmaking services. In cancer, I had become quite adept at figuring out which doctor was the one to go to for what information. I learned the difference between a good match and a bad one. I was able to do the same thing for my fellow law students. One of my favorite activities was matching interns with law practices. Because I had learned the value of speaking up and asking questions, I never hesitated in picking up the phone and asking a firm what they needed and telling them who would be a good fit. In a world of text messages and emails, it amazes me what a simple phone call can do.

I use the same skills now in helping other cancer patients find the right doctors and treatments. When I'm looking at a single problem, the answers become clearer. Chunking it has become an entire lifestyle for me!

# CHAPTER FIVE

# SORRY NOT SORRY

*I was not sorry, nor will I ever be sorry for all those times that I stood up against and irritated frustrated physicians, nurses, and other practitioners whose decisions had a direct impact on my healthcare.*

✦

At times, I think I may just be one of the most insensitive people to ever have entered the cancer community and gone on to become an advocate for others. I've always been pragmatic, driven, and blunt—not out of any malice but simply because I think fast and talk fast and usually move on before checking to see if everyone is caught up.

Cancer culture is filled with optimism—often unreasonable, certainly unbridled, optimism. Inspirational placards, reassuring posters, ribbons and kittens and rainbows, oh my. If optimism could cure cancer, it surely would have by now.

I am not, at heart, an optimist.

Everyone knows someone who has experienced cancer–someone who survived, someone who didn't, someone still fighting. The "cancer culture" is part of our world, for better or worse, and getting a diagnosis dropped me dead-center into the middle of it.

I was surprised at first that when I discussed my diagnosis with family, friends, or even strangers, they would offer personal stories of a loved one or friend, or second cousin's brother who had a similar condition. I understand that this is people's way of relating to me, finding common ground, even commiserating. But these personal stories, despite all good intentions, were often coupled with bad suggestions and misleading information. In an attempt to react in a socially acceptable manner, I had to conceal my real feelings about my diagnosis. I couldn't exactly put my fingers in my ears and sing, "Nah nah nah nah nah, I can't hear you." (Though sometimes I was tempted.) These encounters left me feeling even more overwhelmed and isolated.

When I was diagnosed with stage IV cancer, I didn't turn to *Chicken Soup for the Soul* or inspirational quotes. I turned to science and statistics. These platitudes *can* be very helpful for particular types of people, especially many facing a terminal diagnosis. And I firmly believe that whatever helps the individual in coping and managing illness in the most efficient way, is absolutely the best approach. But when I see a poster of a kitten in a tree and the words "Hang in there!" in an oncology exam room, I want to punch someone (not the kitten, of course. My general frustration with humanity does not extend to animals, no matter how pink the clouds painted behind them).

While I had gone through my life pre-cancer as a direct, strong, indi-vidual—and was pretty consistently treated as such—my cancer diagnosis seemed to try to strip that away. More specifically, the people trying to help me did. Whether it was a doctor who labeled me a difficult, friends who declared me a downer, or family who avoided me, the message was clear. I was no longer Sarah, a person with individual desires, aspirations, and opinions, I was Sarah, cancer patient.

Now, there are *types* of cancer patient I could be. It was socially and medically acceptable to take on the role of cancer warrior in fluffy pink armor or cancer inspiration with a font of platitudes to be doled out whenever a non-cancerous human came within earshot. People were not made uncomfortable if I was the funny cancer patient who cracked jokes about needles and baldness or the wise cancer patient who spoke of God's will and destiny. But these were roles I was to play. Whenever my individuality shone through, it became awkward. But one of the advantages of a terminal diagnosis is getting real real quick. Awkward silence wasn't going to kill me. Asking questions wasn't going to kill me. Pissing people off wasn't going to kill me. Cancer was going to kill me, and it became my only concern.

I was not sorry, nor will I ever be sorry for all those times that I stood up against and irritated frustrated physicians, nurses, and other practitioners whose decisions had a direct impact on my healthcare.

I'm not sorry for how direct I am in my pursuit of the truth and the gritty facts just as they were. I'm not sorry if this takes people aback or offends them.

I have never been a person that has been told or heard that the perception that others have of me is one that is neutral or undecided. To be quite honest, I can't remember a time in my life where I have been told, "Well, I have met her a few times and she seems all right, but I would have to know her a bit more before I could decide."

I tend to be a controversial individual, and I tend to stand firm in the positions that I hold and in my beliefs. Alan Dershowitz told me once that the greatest compliment one could receive is to be un-confirmable. To be un-confirmable means that if I were to be placed in consideration for a position on the Supreme Court that I would undoubtedly not be confirmed. To never take a stand on any issue of controversy in life to the extent that would call for zealous advocacy and relentless strongholds is not a person that I could ever be. After all, if everyone agrees with you, you've made a serious mistake somewhere along the way.

# CHAPTER SIX

# ANOTHER POINT OF VIEW: PETER AND CAITLYNN SMITH ON GRIEF

Maybe because I felt so often that my own perspective was being dismissed, I made a point of trying to understand the perspectives of others. I didn't want to just assume how my cancer was affecting them, so I asked.

This is an interview I conducted with close friends, a husband and wife, Peter and Caitlynn Smith. Peter's experience was one of grief and mourning as he served as his mother's primary caregiver from when she was diagnosed with stage IV breast cancer in 2005 until she passed away in 2008.

**PETER:** My mother died of breast cancer when I was twenty-six years old, and I was her primary caregiver. From the year 2007 to 2008, my mom and I lived at a cancer hospital in Oklahoma: my mother getting experimental treatments and me sleeping on the linoleum every night. When the experimental treatments stopped working, we packed up our bags and moved home to be with my father and brothers.

The hours before my mother's death, approximately eight hours before, I was at home with my mom. She was doing outpatient cancer treatment at the time. That morning she seemed out of it, a little loopy, and we knew something was not right; something was off.

We took her to the emergency room where they conducted a myriad of tests. The tests indicated that my mother had fluid buildup in her lungs, as well as kidney issues. The doctor told us that in order to stabilize her they had two choices. The first option they gave us is that they could give her a particular drug, and if it worked, great. If not, then it was dangerous. The second option was to place my mother on dialysis, which would stabilize her for only a few days, but would give the doctors more time to regroup.

We chose the second option.

By this time, it was late at night, and my father was staying at the hospital. I decided to take my brothers home and sleep for a few hours. I was planning on coming back in the morning, and then I would take it all from there. The phone rang at about two o'clock that morning.

It was my father on the other line, and he was calling from the hospital to tell me that the dialysis treatment had failed, and my mother's condition was not stabilizing. I rushed to the hospital with my brothers, but by the time I'd reached my mother's hospital room she had already passed. I can't tell you how long we spent in the hospital room hugging each other and saying our goodbyes.

When I returned home from the hospital that day there was an overwhelming feeling of sadness with this horrible realization that I would never see my mom wake up in the morning, I would never get the mother and son dance at my wedding—there were no more memories left to be made. The following days morphed into a numbness, a haze, and an inability to feel anything anymore. I think this is partly because of the intensity of the emotions I felt, and I just shut down. I don't remember doing anything those days, what I do remember is that I was in bed barely functioning at a basic level.

**SARAH:** What did you find the most irritating during that time?

**PETER:** When people made some sort of allusion to the fact that God wanted my mom to get better, specifically during my time living in a cancer hospital. I had seen it end tragically for other families and knew the odds of surviving an advanced late-stage diagnosis were not in my mother's favor. Not only that, but how can man presume to know God's will? I was annoyed they made that assumption.

In the end, God chose to take my mother.

I can't remember exactly how much time went by before I talked to people about my mother's death. At first, I was more passive and only communicated through email or text. Then I started talking about it in person. As far as receiving sentiments from other people, one of the initial things was we requested for people not to send flowers or anything like that, but rather make a donation to a charity out of the respect for the type of person that my mother was.

**SARAH:** Did anyone that you had been working with, friends, or family, try to make it better for you?

**PETER:** Most of the support I appreciated because it was passive, but it was respectful, and the way that we had requested. People brought over meals and offered their time, but they gave us space.

**SARAH:** For someone who has lost their parents to cancer, say I have a friend tomorrow who loses her mother, if you could tell that person three things about your experience that you learned that helped you, what would they be?

**PETER:** The first thing is, strange as it may seem, try to accept that as hard as it is, that death is a natural part of life. And that the experience of going through the death of a loved one, in a weird way is a gift that you are given. You don't necessarily have to like it, but it was for me a gift that I learned to appreciate. You can be better off for it; it's made me more appreciative of my friends and family, and I have a greater appreciation for my life and my goals.

The second thing, which is correlated, especially when you're dealing with someone close like a loved one, is that it's essential to the healing process to restore or establish some sense of stability. In the case of losing a parent, they are such a grounding and foundational force in your life, I took on that legacy of being the stabilization and the grounding force for others in my life, and with my loved ones. In essence, that is what I believe is passed on in our parent's legacies. And that is what I tried to take on as part of my mother's legacy.

**SARAH:** There is no way that you would have gotten over it so fast if you did not have a distraction. What was the distraction?

**CAITLYNN:** I was the distraction!

**SARAH:** Tell me about how you pulled that off, Caitlynn, and what helped.

**CAITLYNN:** Well, when I first saw Peter, I was not attracted to him. At all. Peter looked like a forest creature or refugee.

**PETER:** I was depressed after my mother died. I had stopped showering and shaving.

**CAITLYNN:** He wore cargo pants, an army jacket, and tie-dye T-shirts. My friend Kevin took me to his small group Bible study, and I met him there.

After I had met him, I asked Kevin, "Who is your homeless friend?" and Kevin said, "Oh, that's just Peter. He's a great guy."

I started hanging out with the people in the Bible study, many of whom had known each other for years but weren't very close. I kept trying to push the group together and get them to hang out with each other and get to know each other better. As we all grew closer together, I kept trying to get to know Peter because I wanted to be friends with him too.

He would sometimes say that he wanted to go get new clothes and cut his hair. I volunteered to take him to get new clothes because I love to shop, and so this homeless man Peter actually agreed to go shopping with me.

**PETER:** Caitlynn picked me up to take me to the mall, and when I appeared around the corner, I had trimmed my beard and put my hair in a ponytail so that it looked short. And I was in clothes not provided by the Army corps or the Goodwill.

**CAITLYNN:** He looked very handsome!

**PETER:** Caitlynn did not know that my mother had just recently passed until I told her that afternoon, which is why I had been neglecting my looks and cleanliness.

**CAITLYNN:** That afternoon, I got to put Peter in modern clothes, and he looked great! I was starting to think he was really cute.

Later, one of our friends, Stephanie, saw us walking together in the mall and texted me, "Are you out with Peter Smith? You should see the way he looks at you! He's in love!"

The rest of the week, we hung out with each other in a group setting.

**SARAH:** Peter, how did Caitlynn help you as a distraction?

**PETER:** I initially thought that Caitlynn was terrifying. Yet when I met her, it was close to the time that my mom had died, and I was still very introverted and reserved. If it hadn't been for the Bible study, I wouldn't have met or got to know Caitlynn.

The people in the Bible study had been in the church most of their lives as well, but they weren't close friends. They were not people who spent any personal time together outside of the group. When Caitlynn got here, she decided it was her mission to make friends with the people in the Bible study and make them all close friends with each other, too. Now, they are all best friends and roommates!

For me, I took the back way into the Bible study. A long time ago, one of the families that sometimes went to the same church as Kevin was a neighbor, and I ran into them at a restaurant before my mom died. They had invited us to their church, where I heard about the Bible study. It was probably a couple months after my mom died, and I decided to go to Bible study to see if it would help. That is when I contacted this family. I told them that I was interested in attending.

**SARAH:** So Peter was in the Bible study before Caitlynn, and Peter was afraid of butterflies, loud music, bright colors, etc. until he met Caitlynn.

**CAITLYNN:** Then I organized a Bible study bar night.

**SARAH:** Of course, it's Caitlynn that coordinated the Bible study going to bars.

**CAITLYNN.** Peter offered to drive me to the bar, and when he dropped me off, he left me at the curb. To walk down a dark walkway. To say it simply: he had no game.

**PETER:** At this point, we liked each other well enough, but it wasn't working. I was just acting way too weird and was meek as a church mouse. Then the next weekend, I cut my hair, which was so long I was able to donate it to Locks of Love. The rest of the week, we hung out alone before and after group events. Then the following weekend, we went to a party at Caitlynn's beach house. When we were at the beach, knowing I had no game, Caitlynn, to keep my mind off of my mother's death, says, "Are you going to kiss me or what?" and I kissed her. And we've been married for four years.

**CAITLYNN:** Ever since then we have been inseparable!

**SARAH:** Now let's ask Peter about why Caitlynn's personality got him to see outside of his grief. I feel like saying she was "a distraction" is unfair to Caitlynn. I'm a details person, so I want to know what it was about Caitlynn Smith and her really vivacious approach to life that got you to live again, be happy again, get out of that homeless scratch n' sniff garb, and go to a place where you were not afraid of color, my writing, butterflies, stuff like that.

**PETER:** When Caitlynn started coming to Bible study, it was approximately a year after my mother died, and it was when I was beginning to work through things and come out of my shell.

**CAITLYNN:** I think that's a complete lie! You were still so introverted when I got there!

**PETER:** I wanted to stay in the shell, but I was coming out a bit...I decided at this point I needed to start living again.

And I believe now I subconsciously came to that conclusion by watching Caitlynn (who simultaneously terrified and intimidated me). I saw in her this desire to help people in the group become more bonded in their personal lives in a deeper way. Caitlynn connected people in a way that developed meaningful relationships, which I found utterly compelling. I finally wanted to integrate and socialize with the group. I wanted to continue the legacy of my mother through caring for other people and actively being there for people. And here is this crazy woman doing this in her everyday life through her actions.

I saw her as a partner I could spend my life with fulfilling my mom's legacy.

**SARAH:** Caitlynn, were you as perplexed by Peter as he was intimidated and fascinated with you?

**CAITLYNN:** Absolutely, yes! I tried really hard to be friends with Peter because he was part of the crew, but he was still really shy. He rebuffed me! It was all these little things, such as I saw a sign for Peter Street, and I took a picture of the sign and texted it to him. I also sent the message, "Hope you're having a good day!" No response. So I looked up his Facebook profile, and I found out he liked Bobby Darin. I tried to talk to him about Bobby Darin's music, and poor Peter could not name one Bobby Darin song. I walked away from the conversation thinking he was pretentious. But I still wanted Peter to be included in the group (even though I thought that he might be an insane jerk and possibly homeless).

**SARAH:** Therefore, Caitlynn took on the task of properly training you in a way so he was not perceived as a Unabomber, nor as a vagrant wanderer who had lost his mind in the 60s. Knowing Caitlynn, a part of me believes that she saw this as a challenge. So I can see how she would have taken you on, and integrated you, as you would say, into this society of people that you were establishing relationships with. I also believe that Caitlynn did so in the hopes she could figure you out, and you could eventually, like everyone else whose ever had the fortune of coming across Caitlynn in their lives, find her one of the most lovable and endearing people you will ever meet.

**PETER:** Another quality she has is spontaneity, and after my mother's death I was very unlikely to be a person who could say, "Let's jump in the car and go to the beach!" Or decide on the spur of the moment to go for a hike.

It all ties back to living life again, which is something that I completely lost after my mother's death. And with Caitlynn and her zest for life, I started to see what living life after losing my mother could look like for the first time.

I had a newfound curiosity. Even just watching documentaries on something new helped broaden me a little bit, and I appreciated that

Caitlynn brought this to the table. And I also think that Caitlynn's ability to see the best in people was something I loved. She certainly saw the best in me when I was at my worst: looking sad in my tie-dye. I genuinely and sincerely appreciate that she still tried to befriend me despite my outdated fashion choices.

Before my mother died, I tended to be much more judgmental and not understanding of others. Caitlynn had the ability to look at the circumstances and situational context of people and find what was good and pure about everyone. And this is what I love about Caitlynn, and this is what I can say I strive to be a better person for, so that I can be a better person for myself, and be a better person for Caitlynn, and for others. In doing this, I have grown tremendously. Following my mother's death, I stopped taking chances on things that were new to me, even people that were scary at first or intimidated me. And it's Caitlynn who taught me to look again, and to love again.

# CHAPTER SEVEN

# DRUGS

*You're going to come across problems during your cancer treatment that will require all your resources to solve. Your pharmacist is one of your best resources.*

✦

The sheer amount of things that have to be tracked with cancer is staggering. But I had no choice. Understanding prescribed medications and their intended purpose was not only essential in allowing me to take an active role in my health care, but it was also a very real safety concern. Medications can interact with other medications, foods, even non-prescription supplements, and the results can be life-threatening.

While undergoing my second regimen of chemotherapy, one of the treatments was a chemotherapy pill. This pill interacted with tyramine, a chemical commonly found in many food and beverage items. The interaction between the chemotherapy pill and tyramine could cause a life-threating drop in blood pressure. Because of this, I adhered to a very specific diet to prevent this adverse side effect.

From the very beginning of my treatment, I was given high doses of the narcotic painkiller oxycodone (found in Percocet and Oxycontin). Prior to my diagnosis, I had never taken a prescription pain pill in my entire life.

After my first ultrasound, I learned that the pain in my right hip had been so severe because the tumor was pressing up against my sciatic nerve. When I first started treatment, my oncology team told me if I did not "get ahead of the pain" I would be constantly chasing it and would end up taking more and more painkillers. This is a common problem in pain care management. We don't want to take a lot of narcotics, so we take the minimum. That takes the edge off, but the pain comes back before the next dose is due. So we take another—take the edge off—need more, until by the end of the day we've taken more than we would have had we just taken a higher dose at regular intervals. Once the doctor explained this to me, I understood. In theory.

My doctors in Reno, Nevada, prescribed high doses of pain medication in large quantities, but I couldn't keep up with them because they made me so ill. This was during the first few weeks of my diagnosis when I was scared to death of not following my oncologist's instructions to the letter, and I complied.

At that point, the Reno medical team had instilled the fear of God in me that I would suffer terrible pain, even greater than the pain that I had initially felt, and would be in agony if I did not take each and every prescribed pill. The idea that I would be writhing in pain for the rest of my treatment was terrifying. So, I picked up my prescriptions from my Walgreens pharmacist as scheduled, and struggled to take the prescribed dosages every four hours on the dot, twenty-four hours a day. I was miserable.

Between the high dosages of unnecessary pain medication and the chemotherapy, I could barely move from nausea. I curbed my symptoms with a well-known anti-nausea medication, Zofran, which I also I took without fail. At the time, I didn't understand that the high dosages and frequency of the opiates were causing dependency.

It concerns me the ease with which my Reno oncologists wrote prescriptions for such medications, knowing they were highly addictive. It wasn't until later that I realized my oncologist would have little, if any, thought of what the rehabilitation process would look like because I was never meant to live to see that point.

The pain medications were essentially comfort care, and the dosages were not controlled until I reached Stanford Cancer Center. It was there that Dr. Ginna Laport quickly began regulating my dosages and decreasing them. Dr. Laport believed there was a chance I could survive cancer treatment, and she did not want me to come out the other side of treatment with a crippling addiction. For the first time, I had a team of oncologists thinking about the quality of my life—not just the quality of my life at the time—but the quality of my life beyond what it might look like after cancer.

Not only did my team consider this, Dr. Laport incorporated it into my treatment and management of my health care. From the first day, Dr. Laport was set on me living past cancer, in spite of the odds.

In August 2012, I was going through the preparation phase (more chemo, this round a much higher dose) before receiving my bone marrow transplant, when I experienced five days that I can only describe as the most terrifying five days of my life.

Back in July 2012, I had fired my Reno team and was now being treated by Dr. Laport at Stanford. By that time, I had undergone two bone marrow biopsies (including the unsuccessful attempt in Dr. Reese's office), unsuccessful fertility treatments, PowerPort placement, multiple rounds of chemo (ABVD), recurrence of my cancer leading to a more aggressive and higher dose chemo (BEACOPP), and more tests than I could count.

Dr. Laport ordered a PET scan to determine whether or not I was responding to the escalated BEACOPP chemotherapy regimen. It was crucial that my scan show that my cancer was responding to the new chemotherapy, ABVD had failed in May. The only chance at taking a shot at saving my life, which Dr. Reese and Dr. Shefield had given up on months before as a lost cause, was for me to have the bone marrow transplant at Stanford. However, in order for me to have the bone marrow transplant, my cancer would have to show that it was responding to the escalated BEACOPP treatment, because if the transplant were to fail, the fatality rate is 100 percent.

The PET scan showed that my cancer *had* responded sufficiently to the escalated BEACOPP regimen—to the point where Dr. Laport, and the transplant team at Stanford felt that we could proceed with the transplant.

In August, I prepped for transplant with high-dose chemotherapy. This chemotherapy was unlike anything I had ever experienced. Dr. Laport called it "whopping" dosages. It was about eight times the amount of an average chemotherapy infusion.

My first infusion was done in hospital at Stanford, and despite the whopping dosages of chemotherapy I was so happy to be there I actually look back at that first high-dose infusion as a good experience. I had a roommate, and she and I laughed and told cancer war stories. Stanford even had menus, *real* menus with salmon as an option. I did order it once, but I don't remember if I ate it. I am sure if I did it didn't stay down long, but I do remember thinking this is how this whole cancer experience, my cancer experience, should have been the entire time.

This is how is should be for everyone. Between telling each other stories, jokes, and having family visits and trying out every food item on the menu, my roommate and I were very sick, there was no hiding that, but we had fun too, and we laughed. For the first time there were glimpses of bright spots, and it wasn't from an oncoming migraine. This time, it was hope.

Then came the five days from hell.

I had just returned home to the ranch from the Stanford Cancer Center and was given about a week or so before I would need to return to be admitted to the hospital for my bone marrow transplant. Harrison was able to take some time off work and had come to join me and support me as I readied for my transplant. At this point, my system was a cocktail of chemotherapies and prescription drugs.

The combination of all the medications and drugs resulted in an almost complete psychotic and neurological breakdown that lasted the span of five days. I was utterly defenseless against what was happening to my body and my mind. At that point, cancer was no longer what I feared would take my life because, in those five days, the biggest threat to my life was me.

At my last appointment at Stanford before returning home to the ranch, I had been prescribed an antidepressant medication, which is widely used to treat millions of people in the United States today. It was prescribed to me because it had an off-label use for the management of anxiety. At this point during my treatment, I had been on a strict and high-dose pain management treatment plan that included the use of opiates, sleeping medication, and anti-anxiety medications prescribed in addition to transplant doses of chemotherapy.

Almost immediately after taking this medication mixture, I couldn't sit still. My body was trembling, and I felt as if my skin was holding back thousands of insects, clawing and thrashing at each other underneath my skin. For the first day, I tried to get some sleep, and although I was exhausted, I was barely able to lay still, every cell becoming increasingly restless. When it initially started, I kept reminding myself that my doctor had told me I would become irritable and agitated and that it would last for approximately two weeks. If I could get through those two weeks, these symptoms would diminish. I told myself that those symptoms were what I was experiencing.

The first evening, I swallowed the handfuls of pills that I did every night and tried to lay with Harrison in bed and watch a movie. Within an hour or so, my symptoms started, and my mind changed. My thoughts raced; I had an overwhelming sense of dread and anger. I felt as if I had become a mouse trapped in an infinite race, crashing into walls, desperately trying to find an exit.

By the second day, I experienced a profound well of sorrow, which morphed into a crippling depression. I had no idea what was happening to me, and neither did my family. I knew something was seriously wrong, and I reached out almost hourly to my medical team at Stanford as they scurried to find the cause, and a remedy, as my mental anguished soared.

The following morning, my mother found me just before sunrise sitting on the couch, holding myself as I rocked violently back and forth, crying and shifting my feet rapidly. I had spent the entire night alternating between rocking and pacing up and down the stairs.

My body insisted on physically exhausting itself, pushing itself to its physical peak. I could only sit for a few minutes without getting the urge to pace up and down the staircase, like a wind-up toy soldier.

It was at this point that I began to scare my family.

My condition continued to deteriorate despite Harrison, my family, and my medical team's best efforts to help me.

By the fourth day, I reached the breaking point. I hadn't slept for four days. For the first time in my life, I was fighting suicidal impulses as if they were cravings for chocolate cake during Lent.

That day, my doctors had prescribed a new medication, and I had to go along with my mother to pick it up at the Rite Aid because she was scared to leave me alone. I was forced to make that twenty-minute drive with my mom, which was one of the most difficult things I've ever done due to the feeling of wanting to jump out of my skin. Tiny insects clawed at me beneath my flesh, trying to scrape their way out. Given the option of having to take that ride in the car again or having to remove my own fingernails, I'd gladly ask you to hand over the pliers.

We pulled up to the Rite Aid, and as I was rocking back and forth maniacally, trying not to crawl out of my skin, the pharmacist, Dan, collected my prescriptions. He was a very handsome, older gentleman and had always been kind to me.

I couldn't take it anymore. No one could help me, and none of my doctors knew what was wrong. When Dan came to the window and opened it to ask me questions about my prescriptions, I couldn't help myself. I leaned over my mother in the driver seat and asked Dan for help. "Help me," I croaked, unable to even form a question. My mother told him what was happening, what I was experiencing, and how terrified we were because no one could seem to figure out what was wrong with me.

We were desperate at that moment. Reaching out to this pharmacist who was my last hope, my Hail Mary play. Dan had the complete list of medications I had been prescribed, and rather than telling me to call my physician and come back once I had another prescription to fill, Dan took it upon himself to look into it without any delay. I had never actually viewed pharmacists as a crucial resource I could use in the management of my health care, but this man, Dan, proved to be just that.

It was unbelievable. Within ten minutes, Dan had identified exactly what was wrong and precisely what medication had caused it. He was taken aback by the fact that I had been prescribed these medications at the same time as one another. He was aghast that none of my doctors bothered to check with each other to make sure there wouldn't be any detrimental interactions between the medications. It was these drugs that in combination resulted in a pharmaceutically induced psychosis.

Dan instructed me just to stop taking one particular medication entirely. I couldn't believe that the answer was that simple, and I didn't believe it was going to work. My mother asked Dan how long it would take before I regained control of my mental and physical capacities, and I remember him responding that it would happen almost immediately once the medication left my system. Less than twelve hours later that is exactly what happened.

Almost immediately once the medication was out of my system, all of the symptoms subsided, all of the mental and emotional turmoil ceased, and I slept for hours.

For the first time, on the fifth day, my perception of time adjusted back to normal. I can tell you everything that happened during those five days down to the smallest, most minuscule details: what I was wearing, every televisions episode I watched, and the exact times my mother and fiancé went to sleep and woke up. I was fortunate enough to have the foresight to get help wherever I could find it and to ask for it. And I was extremely lucky to have Dan as my pharmacist.

Cancer treatment is all about medications. Lots and lots of medications. And even the best doctors can miss interactions because there is no one person writing all the prescriptions. Because I live in a small town, I only went to one pharmacy, a coincidence for which I am incredibly thankful. Dan was the only person who knew every medication I was on. I had multiple doctors prescribing medications for me, but only one pharmacist filling them all. No matter the size of the town, and regardless of any inconvenience, every cancer patient should find a good pharmacist and then stick with him or her. Having one pharmacist as the hub for all medicinal treatments is a lifesaver.

If you're going through cancer treatment, you are going to come across problems that will require all your resources to solve. Your pharmacist is one of your best resources. He or she is educated specifically on the interactions and chemical makeups of the medications you will be taking throughout treatment. Most of the time the pharmacist knows better than the doctors if there are any potentially detrimental drug interactions between the medications in the treatment plan prescribed. Ever since Dan saved me, I always check with my pharmacist when I have questions about side effects or interactions from the medications I'm prescribed.

# PART TWO

# TAKING BACK CONTROL

# CHAPTER EIGHT

# WHEN GOOD ENOUGH
# MAY GET YOU KILLED

*However, not one of my Reno oncologists informed me that they no longer thought it possible for my cancer to go into remission or even be slowed down: they were all waiting for me die.*

✦

M ay 3, 2012, was the day I became an active patient. Six months of rather uneventful chemotherapy had bought me some time. Then I had an appointment with one of the head oncologists on my medical team in Reno, Nevada, Dr. Reese, because I needed to know whether or not I would be having radiation treatment. I was already exhausted. I had been spending all my time during the previous two weeks or so, working with the University of Connecticut law school to try and get me back into the swing of things and catch up with the rest of the class by taking summer classes. I met with him right before my scheduled chemo (ABVD) infusion. Having done my own research, I knew that the standard of care was that patients who present with "bulky" disease (tumors larger than six centimeters) must receive radiation treatment as part of the protocol. At this point, we were expecting to have the ABVD chemo to have been successful, but Dr. Reese needed to make the call on whether or not I would need to undergo radiation treatment and whether or not I could do it in Connecticut instead of Reno.

I reminded Dr. Reese that my tumor was larger than six centimeters and so I fully expected radiation. The question was where I would have it. But Dr. Reese became very flustered when I wanted to clarify this with him, and immediately he told me that I would not have radiation treatment because my largest tumor was six centimeters.

Without hesitation, I corrected him and politely asked him to pull my file and to review it with me right then because he was seriously mistaken: the tumor was fourteen centimeters. Until this point, I'd been a passive patient, listening quietly, doing what I was told, being a good girl. But I knew he was wrong—not only wrong but wrong on a major component of my disease. Dr. Reese did not respond well to this, and he went storming into the chemotherapy infusion room, me right on his heels (I still had to get chemo) and I asked him again to pull the file as well as his medical notes on my case for me to review. He was infuriated and absolutely insulted that I was suggesting he was wrong and had the audacity to challenge him.

In what would ultimately be the moment that decided my fate, there we were in front of the entire chemo patient infusion room, in what was a clear HIPAA violation, with all the other patients, staff, and doctors as witnesses, Dr. Reese, looked me dead in the face and lost all semblance of professionalism. In what felt like a gauntlet challenge, he said, "Let's settle this once and for all! What are you going to do? Are you going to force me to order a PET scan to prove this to you?" I thought about this for a moment before I responded because that was actually a fantastic idea.

Taking my hesitation as acquiescence, he went straight to his office and shut the door. I was so shocked I started crying and simply sat down for my chemo.

I had been reading Neil Fiore's book *Coping with the Emotional Impact of Cancer* (Bay Tree Publishing, 2009) by this time, and my infusion gave me time to think about what had just happened in light of what I'd been reading. Dr. Reese was exhibiting several red flag behaviors in the management of my care. He was acting not just rushed but frantic and couldn't talk about the issue. When he was asked a question, he became immediately defensive and impatient. This quickly led to an inability to focus on me as a patient. When I cornered him with a question, he gave me political speak—lots of words but no meaning. When I tried to get him to slow down and explain what he was trying to say, he got inpatient and made me feel like I was wasting his valuable time. Even his body language spoke volumes. He wouldn't look me in the eyes and his body remained firmly turned toward the door and away from me. He never even sat down. Most disturbing, in an office that had no electronic systems for patient continuity of care, he never took any notes. He never even opened my file. When things did not go his way and I challenged him, he refused to participate in the conversation any longer or admit he might be wrong.

It was time to stand up and advocate for myself just as Dr. Fiore had mapped out. As soon as my infusion was complete, I demanded that my medical team immediately order a PET scan for the following morning.

I knew after weeks of medically invasive treatments that my tumor was above the threshold needed for radiation treatment, and yet this man, whose hands I had entrusted with my very life, made me feel inferior and ignorant. It was more than just the public shaming and insulting way he treated me, it was that I knew radiation could mean the difference between my life and my death and the callous doctor couldn't be bothered to simply pull a medical chart to double check an essential fact.

I cried all the way through chemotherapy after that interaction, knowing had I not begged for my very survival, if I had blindly let the doctor treat me like a piece of trash billowing in the breeze, my very existence would have been in mortal peril.

I questioned whether Dr. Fiore had gotten it all wrong, and I was the idiot who tried and failed to implement his strategies. The decision I made to stick to the active patient strategy saved my life. Would I have chosen any other actions that day, it would have been a much different outcome. The PET scan would show that my cancer had metastasized 75 percent and if I did not enter treatment that exact day, I would have died. The choices I made that day are the only thing that prevented this oncologist from costing me my life.

✦

## May 4, 2012

I sat with my mother in the claustrophobic exam room when I heard Dr. Reese outside the door creating his typical chaotic working environment.

He came through the door as if fleeing a crime scene. He was frantic, breathing heavily and began to speak very quickly.

The following is from my recording of the appointment:

**DR. REESE:** Sarah, at this point you have failed. I've just gotten off the phone with Stanford and they said you need a chemotherapy called BEACOPP, escalated BEACOPP. Dr. Advani [Stanford] says that for those who don't do good on ABVD, and it fails for some patients who are then randomized to escalated BEACOPP. There will definitely be a bone marrow transplant if there is success with within the first two cycles [four weeks] BEACOPP. This is a much higher intense chemotherapy, much higher toxicity. The side effects are increased nausea, vomiting, loose stools , heart and lung toxicity, which will be checked through pulmonary function test.

**SARAH:** So I will be having a transplant?

**DR. REESE:** You need transplant for sure, and this will definitely be done at Stanford. We need to start the BEACOPP tomorrow at the latest. You will not be able to return to school this year.

**SARAH:** Should Harrison move back?

**DR. REESE:** It is your personal choice.

**SARAH:** What are the chances it won't work?

**DR.REESE: Always** 50/50 chance.

**SARAH:** With how fast the tumors are growing what is my prognosis?

**DR. REESE:** The radiologist is very concerned about new spots on the spleen and on the liver. What I am going to do is admit you now to the hospital; we are just waiting for a room.

**SARAH:** If the BEACOPP fails, how long do I have to live?

[*Dr. Reese says nothing.*]

**SARAH:** A year...?

[*Dr. Reese says nothing*]

**SARAH:** Six months...?

**DR. REESE:** At best

When I listen to the recordings of the doctor's appointments from those days, they're frantic and furious. They're chaotic and confusing. It became clearly evident that I was far out of the depths that my team of oncologists at the time could handle in a competent manner. In what took the cancer cells several years to metastasize into had adapted and rapidly morphed, riddling my body with hundreds of tumors in just three short months.

Once again, my time was running out fast, and I was locked in a dead race to try and save my life. It was one of the rare moments in my life when tough decisions had to be made and my emotional responses, as difficult as they were to put aside, became irrelevant. I didn't have time to feel those emotions. Every decision my medical team, in Reno, would make became a matter of life or death. My death.

I finally fired Dr. Reese, and Dr. Shefield took over my care.

There was one last hope to save my life, and it began with the restaging and induction of the German chemotherapy regimen, BEACOPP, in its most aggressive combination, referred to as escalated BEACOPP. It is from this point forward that I faced my darkest hours, wrestled with my mortality, and ultimately reconciled my past with my present state, letting go of what I had once thought my life would be, and reaching a place where I was no longer afraid of death and viewed my mortality with eyes wide open.

✦

By June, my health was declining so quickly that I was beginning to receive palliative care in Reno. However, not one of my oncologists informed me that they no longer thought it possible for my cancer to go into remission or even be slowed down: they were all waiting for me die. I finally realized it when a late-night conversation with a nurse led me to ask how many people were designated terminal on the cancer floor I had been assigned, and the only thing she said was, "everyone."

I was twenty-four years old, on my deathbed, and I wasted no more time. I called an emergency meeting with my medical team right then, in the middle of the night. Everyone from the social worker, the oncology nurse, the physicians assistant, even the head of the hematology center, met in my room. I sat them down all around my hospital bed and I had them tell me face to face that they were no longer pursuing treatment, but now just making my time left comfortable.

"Dr. Shefield, do you believe in my survival?"

"No," Dr. Shefield replied in an abrupt indifferent response. "You will never see a courtroom again, you will never study law again. Stop this and spend the rest of the time you have with your family."

Knowing it would mean getting rid of the entire oncology team, I fired Dr. Shefield. I demanded that she call the Stanford Cancer Center, and make the referral immediately.

Stanford Cancer Center took me on as a patient the next day, and I was given a team of the best lymphoma oncologists in the world. Once my care was transferred, I found out Dr. Reese had been lying to me. He had told me that Stanford refused my care. I now found out they had been following my case since the beginning. It was Dr. Reese who had refused the transfer, noting in my medical chart that he had given me the option of doing a clinical trial at Stanford and that I refused. This broke my heart when my medical records were finally released to me from this oncology practice in 2015. After listening repeatedly to the recordings of those appointments with Dr. Reese and hearing him tell me and my mother when we specifically asked to go to Stanford that we would not be accepted, and then to read these lies noted in my medical chart was just further confirmation of his callousness. It still hurt.

Nevada currently ranks 48th out of the 50 states in terms of oncology care and the quality of practitioners. That's a pretty dry statistic, one I knew about before I began treatment. But I think it's natural to think, "Sure, but not my doctor." I don't know if it's wishful thinking or denial, but I've talked to many other people now who were unwilling to think their own doctors were less than the best, often despite all evidence to the contrary.

That night, listening to a group of medical professionals tell me they didn't even entertain the possibility of my surviving treatment woke me up and spurred me into action.

# CHAPTER NINE

# SEEING RED

*Mediocrity can be countered through the increased role you play in your health-care, taking on the role of the researcher and cross referencing what you're told directly from your physician with studies, research, and online communities.*

✦

Sometimes I imagine what it would've been like to be one of the Confederate soldiers during Pickett's Charge up Cemetery Hill during the Battle of Gettysburg. In following orders, the soldiers were lead directly to their graves. I am assuming that in the majority of the cases, by the time they entered the open meadow and realized the dire mistake their leaders had made, it was too late. It was too late for them to question the tactical decisions and strategies; it was too late to stop and try to regain the ground that had been lost because to stop would result in almost certain death. It was too late for any of them to do anything except to take another step and try to dodge the cannon fire from 160 Union cannons. It was up to each man to try and stay alive by judging for himself what the best course of action would be to get across more than 5,000 feet of open meadow. The soldiers became responsible for their own lives as they entered the open area, and if they were to survive they needed to take an active role in every step they took after that moment.

How can we identify a red flag if we do not understand what to look for? How can we question our leaders, and our doctors if we don't know what the issues are? How as cancer patients can we guard against blindly following an oncologist or a treatment plan, which unbeknownst to us is faulty? How do we prevent ourselves from walking into the open meadow before it is too late?

Hindsight is 20/20. So I suggest that unless you want to be crossing a figurative 5,577-foot stretch of meadow under fire, pay attention and note your intuition, as it will likely save your life at some point. Do not second-guess yourself if you believe that you have identified a crucial red flag. Cancer treatment is black-and-white, and it pays to always, without a doubt, assume nothing and question everything.

The next time you feel that the questions you have written down or issues that arise during an appointment are secondary or irrelevant, just remember Cemetery Ridge and what happened to the soldiers in Pickett's Charge. Don't place yourself in the meadow if you don't have to.

Though it took extremely obvious red flags for me to take action in my care, every red flag is critical. I've seen the most seemingly meaningless question save a life, the most extreme stance against accepted practices turn the tide, and the most random interventions become miracles. I've also seen stubbornness result in death, well-meaning friends derail a successful course of treatment, and denial eat up valuable time. In each case, with hindsight and honesty, the patient knew the truth. Whether it was taking the unexpected path or staying in step, they each knew in their gut which way to go. The best you can do for yourself is be honest. Cancer treatment is no place for egos.

I can not stress strongly enough the importance of having quality communications with doctors. Let me switch gears a little to bring this point home.

The following two stories demonstrate some common mistakes that are made during cancer treatment by doctors and patients. Place yourself in both Sally and my shoes. Take a few minutes after reading each to check in with your gut. What would you do in these two circumstances?

*Sally was a new patient and was diagnosed with stage IV non-Hodgkin lymphoma. Sally was 49 years old at the time, and had never had any cancer-related issues prior to her diagnosis. Sally lived in a mid-sized town with a population of roughly 500,000 people, two hospitals, and about fifteen primary oncologists to choose from, three of which specialized in her particular cancer. Sally chose to go to the specialist who had the most extensive experience in treating her type of cancer and had the most practical experience in terms of years practicing oncology. Sally attended her first appointment with her new primary oncologist, who was a fifty-seven-year-old white male, who lead the oncology practice from which Sally would receive treatment.*

One of the most challenging and identifiable potential red flags is the limited amount of medical resources available to Sally in her mid-sized town. However, to offset the extent of the impact of the limited medical resources, prior to selecting an oncologist, Sally could have utilized the technological resources that are available such as online reviews of hospitals and doctors.

The second issue is generational. Here, we have two people from a generation that operates under the traditional physician-centered model. In this traditional model, technological innovations and advancements are not taken into consideration, particularly because they have only recently reached a level where they are being utilized to shift medicine to a patient-centered framework. Without these technological advancements, the traditional model, under which the oncologist has presumably been practicing for more than twenty years, treats the physician as the ultimate authority. The patient is expected to defer to the physician for expertise and guidance on most, if not all, treatment matters. The patient's role is a peripheral one. Only recently, within the past ten years or so, has this dynamic begun to change.

While, it is true that some patients while coping with the diagnosis of cancer will become too overwhelmed to play an active role in their medical care and decisions (been there, done that), it is important to get past that. Patients always have the right to ask questions, ask for clarity on issues, and seek second opinions if they have reservations. I learned this lesson after my first chemotherapy failed and my primary oncologist had given me a ten percent chance for survival. Rather than accept this prognosis, I sought a second opinion from Stanford, where I was given a life-saving bone marrow transplant. This decision saved my life, but it took backing me into a corner for me to make it. We all have the right to seek a second or third opinion, and to find doctors who we feel are ALWAYS acting in our best interest, and provide the most up-to-date medical treatments.

Sally would be wise to look for behavioral indicators such as inattentiveness, passive listening, being interrupted by the physician when speaking, a sense of unrest or time constraints placed on the appointment by the physician, and perhaps most importantly, whether or not in the initial appointment the physician asks Sally about her emotional and mental well-being. This is important because it is indicative that the physician is addressing key psycho-social factors outside of Sally's technical diagnosis that are key to her overall health and well-being.

*Sally scheduled her first appointment, and unfortunately it was a chaotic time of year as Sally was diagnosed right around Christmas. Throughout the process of the determination of whether or not Sally's biopsy was, in fact, cancerous, and then moving on to the staging, and identification of the particular type of cancer, Sally was told multiple times by several attending doctors and nurses at the hospital where the procedures were performed that beginning a treatment plan as soon as possible was imperative to the success of the treatment. Sally knew that if she delayed treatment past the holiday season, it could cost her her life. But when Sally called to schedule her first appointment with her new primary oncologist, she was told that the office would be closed for the holidays and that her physician would be on leave. However, they could get Sally in as soon as possible after the first of the year. Sally went ahead and made an appointment for January second.*

First, imagine that you're Sally. You have been diagnosed with terminal cancer and have been forced to schedule the start of your treatment after the holiday season even though you know this could be detrimental to your health. But what could she do? Plenty.

It is never, in any situation or circumstance, acceptable for a cancer patient to have to work around the holiday schedule whether it is Christmas, Thanksgiving, or Labor Day. Cancer never takes a holiday; it doesn't have a smartphone to reschedule and plan around other people's schedules when it chooses to metastasize. No physician's holiday is more important than a person's healthcare. No one should be in a situation where cancer is working away, but the doctor is on vacation. This is a serious red flag.

There are at least three ways to handle this sort of scheduling dilemma, none of which delay treatment. First, the patient can ask the doctor's office to refer him or her to another practice that has immediate openings. Second, the patient could try and make an appointment with a larger hospital or practice where there are more doctors on staff. Third, the patient can simply push. In medicine, the squeaky wheel does indeed get the grease. While there is never cause to be rude, remarkable things happen when a patient is firm about his or her needs. This is especially true during the holidays, when everyone is busy and it is easy for someone in scheduling to simply not be aware of the importance of fast action.

*After thinking about her options, Sally called back and politely but firmly demanded that she receive proper care. She was able to get an appointment the next day rather than having to wait until January second.*

*At the first appointment, Sally met her new primary oncologist. Sally had written down a number of questions that were relatively generic and that come up in several frequently asked questions searches on WebMD. It was forty-five minutes after her scheduled check-in time before she was called back by one of the nurses, going back and forth in her mind how she wanted to phrase her questions, trying to calm her nerves. She was placed in one of the small rooms and took a seat on the examination table, where the nurse left her. Another fifteen minutes passed before an older gentleman came swiftly into the room, pulled out a black swivel chair from under the desk, and sat down in one sweeping motion. Immediately he looked at Sally and began writing in her medical chart. The physician then told Sally to lie down, as he would like to take her vitals. He took her blood pressure, temperature, and began pressing around the outside of her neck as well as on both sides of her stomach and lower abdomen.*

*While doing this, the physician said nothing to Sally other than tell her when she could sit up after he examined her. The doctor wrote down some notes in Sally's medical record and told her that he would like to ask her a couple of questions. At this point, Sally was thinking that he was going to make some sort of connection on a personal level with her as his patient. Rather, the physician pulled out an extensive symptoms checklist and ran through the list, word for word. Once he was done with the checklist, the doctor looked at Sally and explained that he would be putting her on a regimen that would include chemotherapy and radiation, which he would like for her to start the next day.*

*The physician then looked at Sally, smiled, and asked her if there was anything else or if she had any questions for him. Sally was completely overwhelmed and did not know where to start. She crumpled up the list she had gathered. She quickly slumped into a passive patient disposition, and asked only one question, "What time do I need to be here tomorrow morning?"*

Since beginning to work with cancer patients, I have read and thoroughly analyzed several top hospitals' and cancer centers' best practice guidelines in dealing with patients. What I have found has been both encouraging and also very disappointing. What distinguishes the mediocre practices and facilities from those at the top of the field is the way that the medical appointments are structured. As we see in the last part of Sally's story, Sally was not given deference or the opportunity to ask even the simplest questions until after she had been hit with the one-two punch of her diagnosis and having to start treatment the next day. Even for the most assertive of us, it can be difficult when we are first diagnosed and our physician appears to be very busy. The doctor is working diligently to make sure that he has all the information he needs, even if we have no idea what the information is and why it is relevant. We assume that the questions that the physician asks of us are more relevant, and the ones we most desire to have answered, such as those concerning the psychosocial aspects of treatment, are secondary. Additionally, we feel indebted to our physicians for the time they spend asking questions on our case, and we don't want to burden them with questions they do not feel are relevant. We act as if the doctors are doing us a favor, rather than acting as if they are providing a professional service for which we are paying.

It is common for physicians, especially those who have been in practice for twenty or more years, to set up patient appointments in a way that makes it difficult for the patient to get the opportunity to ask too many questions. This dynamic is not an accident. It is designed for efficiency for the medical team, to maximize billings and keep up with the workload necessary to sustain a practice. When a physician is controlling the dynamic between him or herself and the patient in a way that discourages questions, that is a serious red flag. It is not uncommon for a physician to use techniques to guard against any unforeseeable questions in which the physician may not know the answer. They will wait until the end of an appointment to quickly ask if there's anything else or any questions the patient has. At this point, the physician is now standing and no longer sitting, as this is a display of body language, indicating that the doctor only has a relatively short amount of time to discuss the patient's questions before having to move on to the next appointment.

The only physicians who do not encourage or take an active interest in patient questions, regardless of whether or not the doctor sees the questions as relevant for their purposes, are the physicians who are substandard or merely average. Now, I understand that the majority of patients do not have access to the best facilities or specialists in the world, and in most cases, it's not necessary to be treated by the top oncologists in a particular cancer, but it is absolutely essential that any patient in a position like Sally's understand that mediocrity can be countered through the increased role the patient plays in his or her healthcare, taking on the role of the researcher and cross referencing what he or she is being told directly from the physician with studies, research, and knowledgeable online communities.

The following transcription is from an appointment with the head of the oncology clinic where I was initially treated. Thank goodness my mother was there. This was the second appointment I had with this particular physician, after I'd been seeing Dr. Reese for treatment for months. By that point, I had had batteries of tests, a port implanted, bone marrow biopsies and several rounds of chemo. Read the transcript carefully, and think about how you feel this appointment went. After, take a moment to contemplate and even take note, if you would like, of anything that stuck out to you. Then ask yourself why any particular aspect stood out among the rest, and if this were the head of your medical team, what, if anything, would you do?

Dr. Shefield first meeting appointment transcription:

**DR. SHEFIELD:** So, uh, they'll have to print those out for you. Your hemoglobin is 1.1. I mean your white count is 1,200. All these appear to be granule sites. All these appear to be granule sites, which is good, so you're not less than 1,000 granule sites, which is good, so you're not less than 1,000 granule sites. At least that's what the computer says. And your hemoglobin dropped a little bit, 9.4, and your platelet count is 252,000. So we are going to give you the Bleomycin and the Vincristine today, and then... did we also start you on the Neupogen here today? Is that usually what we do?

**MOM:** I think we go to the hospital twenty-four hours after the chemo.

**DR. SHEFIELD:** Well, this is a little different because these are not really mild suppressive agents. That's why we do it now with the low...

**MOM:** And then from here on that's why we go to Carson Valley Hospital?

**DOCTOR SHEFIELD:** Yeah, so I will tell them that they also need to get you a Neupogen shot.

**SARAH:** [mumbles] I don't know if that's ordinary.

**DOCTOR SHEFIELD:** Um, yeah, so, and then you are going to be on that and you get regular blood counts down there and they will tell us what they are, and you basically stay on the Neupogen every day until your white counts gets over 13,000.

**SARAH:** Yeah, that's the number we used last time. I wonder if it was 26,000 last time?

**DOCTOR SHEFIELD:** Yeah, about 26,000. Then you are scheduled for a PET scan on the twelfth.

**MOM:** We are!

**DOCTOR SHEFIELD:** Are you? That's what you told me, but I have no idea what you are scheduled for.

**MOM:** Because she's got that follicle extraction, so it's in between the eleventh and the thirteenth, but we don't know when she is going to have to have the [follicle] retrieval. So we are not sure when the PET scan is. But my question is since she is going to, can we do the PET scan up here when she's on the prednisone?

**DOCTOR SHEFIELD:** You mean the Neupogen?

**MOM:** The prednisone, because she's on the prednisone for fourteen days. So should we wait?

**DOCTOR SHEFIELD:** It's probably a little bit better if we wait to see, then it would be nice... [mumbles] because it will probably show... but that's OK. Really what we're looking at is her liver. It will probably be a little better to wait a little bit. I would probably go ahead and let's schedule it for the twelfth. Let's just tentatively schedule it for the twelfth. I think that's a little bit safer to do, and let's just see what you can do as far as the retrievals.

**MOM:** It might be there, but if they have to wait they can always do it there and we can wait and go the next day.

**DOCTOR SHEFIELD:** Yes, you can always do it the next day. How are you doing? Are you all right?

**SARAH:** Yes, I am. Steroids make me a bit puffy, but that's all right.

**DOCTOR SHEFIELD:** Yes, that's part of it.

**SARAH:** We just have a couple questions. The first one was with the Stanford consult; we are going to be going down after the next BEACOPP session. And is that going to happen after, say, the second or third week after I am done with the prednisone? After my counts are the highest?

**DOCTOR SHEFIELD:** Yes, well, we want you to be safe. With your counts up by the time we send you down there.

**SARAH:** The liver numbers, did we run any numbers with the liver today?

**DOCTOR SHEFIELD:** No, we didn't. We sent them out. And we should have them in by tomorrow.

**SARAH:** But the rest of the blood numbers are good?

**DOCTOR SHEFIELD:** Yeah, they do. The important things are that your platelet count is normal. But all this is not unusual. Really, your hemoglobin is 9.4; you have been in that same position. You won't have a problem with that. That will be OK.

**SARAH:** The next question I had is one of the chemotherapies Dr. Reese was saying is toxic and there is a maximum amount you can take during your lifetime. Where am I with that? He said I am only cleared for two more cycles?

**DOCTOR SHEFIELD:** Well, that is, um. Yeah that's the Adriamycin, and I think with that we are going to have to watch that carefully. We will total up the dose to see how much she has had. We do want to be careful with that. I don't think she is close to anything there. I think she is OK.

**SARAH:** Oh, good. At this point, how many cycles of BEACOPP are we expecting? Dr. Reese mentioned four to six and possibly eight, so how many cycles are we expecting?

**DOCTOR SHEFIELD:** Well I think probably four, but it will depend on whether we get a good response. And then we need to talk to Stanford to see what they feel in terms of setting you up to get a transplant. And that's really what we need to know from them.

**SARAH:** And then when we go down to Stanford, are they going to collect the cells for the transplant then, or are they going to use the ones from when I was first diagnosed.

**MOM:** We were just confused about that. She was under the impression that they already took samples when they started in January.

**DOCTOR SHEFIELD:** Oh, no, no. The stem cells that they will take on you, they don't take it from your bone marrow. They do it from the peripheral blood. There are cells from your peripheral blood that they can collect. They hook you up to a machine and they spin those cells and they put everything back in. We used to have to put the patients under anesthesia but that was something like thirty years ago. Now it's much easier. That's a process of wanting to get your blood count up. You're on the Neupogen to get your white count up as high as possible. So we will need to talk to them about coordinating that. Because if we have you on the Neupogen after the BEACOPP it would be nice to be able to do that while you're down there. We have to see if we can work that out. But we have to see after your third one. But we will see what this PET scan shows. That will be important in making a decision about where you are at.

**SARAH:** Now, if the PET scan is not ideally where we want it to be, are we still going to go ahead and move forward and talk with the bone marrow transplant team?

**DOCTOR SHEFIELD:** We will talk to them about where we are at this point, but a lot of it depends on what we see. Hopefully we are going to see a response but the question is how much response. And how much they would want to see before they would want to continue. We know the patients do best if you have the most complete response possible. So that's what we want to achieve

**SARAH:** So that's what we are doing with the BEACOPP? The chemotherapy I will have right before the bone marrow transplant? This is what will get as complete of a response as possible, correct?

**DOCTOR SHEFIELD:** We will talk to them and see if we see a good response, and we will try to consolidate that because even if you can't see anything, there might be microscopic amounts of cells. While we are beating it down we want to continue to beat it down if it's working to give you the best chance for the transplant. And it's really an autologous stem cell transplant. We will use your own cells.

**SARAH:** Those are all my questions.

**DOCTOR SHEFIELD:** We will schedule your PET scan for the twelfth. We are usually able to get it back pretty quickly. If we get it in the morning we can see you in the afternoon.

There are several identifiable red flags at this point. However, while the examples in this chapter are littered with concerning issues, there is essentially one root cause for all of them: mediocrity.

Every single part of this appointment is designed intentionally and shows examples of crucial red flags indicating that mediocrity exists in some critical area. The only physicians who do not encourage or take an active interest in patient questions, regardless of whether or not the doctor sees the questions as relevant for their purposes, are the physicians who are merely average. Now, I understand that the majority of patients do not have access to the best facilities or specialists in the world, and in most cases it's not necessary to be treated by the top oncologists in your particular cancer, but it is absolutely essential that if you are in a position like Sally's mediocrity can be countered through the increased role you play in your healthcare, taking on the role of the researcher and cross referencing what you're told directly from your physician with studies, research, and online communities.

The next time you feel that the questions you have written down or issues that arise during an appointment are secondary or irrelevant, just remember Cemetery Ridge and what happened to the soldiers in Pickett's Charge. Don't place yourself in the meadow if you don't have to.

✦

Not all red flags come from the physicians themselves. Sometimes, their mediocrity shows in the company they keep. I anticipate that while you read this, you'll be thinking to yourself, "clearly Sarah should have seen that as a huge red flag!" But these things weren't quite as apparent when I was in the thick of treatment. Hindsight, again, for the win

As a cancer patient, there is a strong probability that at some point you will be asked if during one of your appointments or consultations a medical student or intern may sit in. If you consent (and you don't have to), use the opportunity to gather information on the practice by simply analyzing the company they keep.

Take note of the intern, the intern's appearance, disposition, and professionalism, as it will be one of the most accurate reflections of your physician's reputation among the medical community. Essentially, ask yourself this question: did your intern "suit-up?" If your answer is "no," it's time to ship out.

Dr. Reese had an intern in the spring of 2012. I was asked if I would consent to have this young female intern sit in on our appointments for educational purposes. This intern was a medical student at the local university, the same university where I received my undergraduate degree. I am all for learning, so I agreed; after all, anything to teach a young doctor. However, what walked through that door following my signature on the consent form, was most assuredly not a young doctor. For a moment, I half expected Ashton Kutcher to pounce from the dark corner of the room and scream, "Punked!" No such luck. This was actually happening.

I was sitting on the examination table when this young intern casually strutted into the room. She plopped down into the chair in the corner, wearing torn jeans and a midriff-baring shirt. When I looked to her feet, I was horrified to see she was wearing flip-flops. In the medical center. I can't tell you what Dr. Reese said that entire appointment, because I was too busy just staring in absolute disgust at this intern's appalling half-chipped-off ratty, dirty toenail polish screaming out from those dirty purple flip-flops. To make matters even more interesting, (and partly the reason why I forgot to start my recording that day), in this tiny room with the four of us, the intern, as if no one would notice, became quickly disengaged and began text messaging.

OMG.

Dr. Reese was clearly more interested in attempting to impress this young standard of excellence with an awkward bedside manner involving the two of us and some hugs that lasted a bit too long. It was a charade; I was offended. I was utterly perplexed that Dr. Reese had allowed an intern in that condition, and without hesitation, to engage with his patients (or more precisely, her phone, in front of the patient). In the end, in doing so, while it showed poorly upon the intern, it spoke volumes about Dr. Reese himself.

I rescinded my consent for any of Dr. Reese's future interns, it was just too much like Forrest Gump and the classic quote, "Life is like a box of chocolates, you never know what you're going to get." I needed to know I was always going to deal with professionals.

Now, at this point, I had met several other interns before this particular gem at several of my other doctor's offices. I was a hot topic that year, because of the rarity and aggressiveness of my cancer, and because my case touched upon just about every oncology specialization out there. The difference between these other interns and Dr. Reese's was night and day.

One of the most impressive interns sat in on my fertility appointment in May 2012. This young woman named Kelsey was well groomed; she had on respectable shoes (which any woman who has been in any type of profession knows, decent shoes are important in the workplace), and she wore a white lab coat. She very quietly smiled, introduced herself, and then sat down in the chair in the corner. She listened diligently and took precise notes. There was nothing distracting about this intern. In fact, I was happy she was there. It was an excellent opportunity for her to learn about fertility in cancer, and she was genuinely interested. She had respect for the physicians that with whom she was working, and she had respect for me as a patient. That signaled to me that she was a person worth my respect. I still think about that intern, and I see a bright future for her.

The intern that the physician has taken on will be a direct reflection of the practitioners themselves. Imagine you are a doctor or a CEO of a small company. Pick an intern. Are we going with door number one, or door number two? What impression would you want to give of your business?

When looking for red flags, gather any information you can from any source you can. And when people show you who they are, believe them.

# CHAPTER TEN

# ON COMMUNICATION

*Alyce never left me, or looked at me any differently than she had when we were young, riding our horses through the hills, racing back, late for dinner, galloping into the sunset.*

✦

Communication about cancer can be complicated, difficult, and can often result in unintended consequences, reactions, and misinterpretations. Knowing how to handle these conversations correctly is crucial for productive, honest, and fulfilling communication throughout cancer treatment. But how do you know how to handle something so foreign?

✦

I noticed two ways people chose to communicate with me: one was by elevating my cancer and one was by seemingly forgetting it. Both were noticeable, but I couldn't predict from day to day, hour to hour, how any comment would affect me.

I remember a time when a close male friend was telling me about his chemo-caused hair loss. He has short close-cropped hair and he was going on at length about how traumatizing it had been to lose it. At the time, my hair had grown back so it was easy to forget what I'd been through. He had. I listened for a solid half hour. I didn't begrudge him his own trauma; I just found it interesting. My own hair loss had not even been in the top ten of the worst things about cancer.

At the same time, I often have people begin or end stories to me with, "Of course, it's nothing like what you went through." While that may be true, it doesn't mean the other person hasn't suffered. While their cancer may have been at an earlier stage or hadn't been terminal, that doesn't mean it wasn't just as traumatic to them. I know that.

Sometimes it really bothers me when people say this. I know they are just trying to be considerate, but sometimes it makes me feel as if I am nothing more than my cancer. That I am only a person relative to cancer. Other times I scarcely notice it.

Some days, I would get offended when people didn't acknowledge how bad my cancer was. Other days, I didn't want people to see the cancer at all. I had good days and bad days.

I found the best way to communicate was to be honest, even if I contradicted myself day to day. I was honest about what I felt in the moment. It helped people around me not worry about hurting my feelings, because they knew that if they did I would tell them. They didn't have to guess.

How you feel about something is always going to come out in your body language anyway. Your tone, your actions—your feelings will reveal themselves.

There is no way to prepare or plan for how to deal with something as singular as stage IV cancer. Nothing quite prepares a person for it. And it's going to change. It is unpredictable and mercurial.

If I wanted people to be honest with me (and I did), I needed to be honest with them. They were watching me for cues. None of my family or friends had been through anything like this either. We were all in unfamiliar territory, and whether I wanted to be or not, I was leading the way.

✦

In law school, I learned about the interest-based approach to communication (based largely on *Getting to Yes: Negotiating Agreement Without Giving In* by Roger Fisher, Penguin Books, 1991). At the time, it seemed just another way of working within the legal system, but it proved crucial in working with the medical field as well.

The interest-based approach to communication is one of the most useful frameworks for communicating about difficult topics when each party has an interest in the outcome. These interests are typically governed by what we look at as the most fundamental human interests—security, economic well-being, sense of belonging, recognition, and control over one's own life.

The interest-based approach to communication begins with identifying one's particular interests and the outcome desired. Once interests have been identified, the next step is to separate the parties from the problem or conflict that is at the center of the difficult conversation. There is a difference between being hard on a problem or issue and being hard on someone with whom you are communicating.

The party who has initiated the conversation should not frame the communication around what has taken place in the past. Instead, he or she should frame the conversation in a way that is not accusatory, nor suggests blame on the other party for the current situation. Rather than focusing on past events, one needs to look toward the future. This will help prevent the other party from feeling he or she is being blamed and avoids the person becoming overly defensive. When individuals become defensive during an awkward conversation, the interest shifts from finding a solution to the problem to fending off what feels like an attack.

It's important that while you maintain a firm stance on where your interests lie and look forward toward a solution, you communicate in a way where you are consistently "soft" on the people and "hard" on the problem.

✦

When it comes to discussing terminal illness, emotions run high. It's inevitable. But emotions can cause us to be irrational and to speak without care and sensitivity, which could result in failure of communication in its entirety.

When going into a difficult conversation, it is imperative to keep your emotions under control. I find the best way to do this is to remember that I am not the only person affected by the conflict or the issue under discussion. I may be the one with cancer, but I am not the only one affected by it. Additionally, it is important for me to remember the impact that my words, behaviors, and attitudes have on those with whom I'm having a conversation. Conversations I never would've thought twice about just a year prior to my diagnosis were now filled with landmines. My illness colored everything I said—and everything I heard.

Often when we are dealing with difficult conversations or topics such as cancer, the people with whom we are engaging are our closest loved ones, our medical or support teams, and those assisting us in financial and insurance matters.

Effective communication is best done by a rational mind where emotions are not completely restrained but are controlled, so as to not let the situation or conversation get out of hand.

Before you begin speaking in a conversation, it's important to look and listen carefully to the person with whom you are talking to try to get a sense of the emotions he or she is bringing to the conversation. If you can identify the other party's interests and the motivating factors behind his or her position, then you will be in the best place to reach an adequate solution.

When you're having a conversation about a topic that does arouse high amounts of emotion, it's important to let the other party discuss with you freely and openly his or her perception of the issue. Don't preach, but rather take the time to really listen and hear what the other party is saying.

Do not be judgmental when someone is openly communicating with you, whether or not you find his or her reasoning to be sound. Should the other party act emotionally, irrationally, or in a particular way that is counterproductive to achieving effective communication, it is important that you maintain your disposition and continue to deal with the other party and act as rationally and level-headed as possible.

Listening to what the other party is trying to say requires active listening rather than passive listening. Active listening requires attention on two levels: first on an intellectual level, which is listening to the message and rationally processing what is being said; the second level is the more intuitive, emotional nuances that help you interpret and listen to the feelings of the other party. Active listening requires patience.

To ensure that you have fully understood what the other person is trying to convey, take a three-second pause between the finish of his or her statements and your response. When we interrupt the other party in a difficult conversation, this can easily give rise to emotional conflicts, which are counterproductive. You'll find that the most successful conversations are a result of listening rather than talking.

Many people have the misconception that active listening and acknowledging the point of the other party means consent or conceding the point. This is not the case. Recognizing the other party's interests and feelings on an issue is different from agreeing with it.

It all boils down to respect. It is important to acknowledge the other side out of respect as a colleague, caregiver, loved one, or another close party. It's important that the person with whom you are speaking knows that you understand his or her position and that you have taken into consideration what it is like to stand in his or her shoes. Both parties will feel mutually respected and feel that their concerns have been heard. Keep in mind that in the end, what matters is that you have reached a satisfactory resolution to a difficult conversation.

When a patient is diagnosed and discusses his or her diagnosis with family and friends, it is likely that he or she will be met with an unexpected reaction from one or two people. This unexpected reaction may cause the patient to experience feelings of guilt or to feel burdensome. This in turn can lower the self-esteem of the patient, which can lead to other issues such as self-isolation and depression. If a patient talks of feelings of guilt or being a burden, it is important to address this issue. Patients need to be aware that people will deal with their cancer diagnosis in differing, sometimes unexpected ways. Relationships may change, and some people may not have the mental or physical capacity to maintain the relationship as it once was.

I ask myself and other cancer patients, "If you had the opportunity for someone to hand you a one-page guide of the top-ten things you should know, what would be on that list?"

On the top of my list would be expecting adverse, strange, and unexpected reactions from the people I thought would be supportive and be by my side the most. Unexpected reactions from the people closest to me struck me hard. That was a pain I was not expecting, and I continue to struggle with it today. But I've come to understand it.

Cancer will change relationships, with some for the better and some for the worse. For the most part, the reactions that I received from family, friends, and even those with whom I had nothing more than a passing acquaintance surprised me. For example, when I discussed my diagnosis with my family and friends, there were individuals with whom I previously had strong relationships who became emotionally isolated and were physically unavailable despite living only minutes away. However, not all unexpected reactions were necessarily bad. Harrison's aunt, for example, whom I had met only once prior to my diagnosis, wrote me encouraging letters and beautiful cards every week.

It is important not to take another's reaction to your cancer diagnosis as a reflection of how the person feels about you. Ultimately, I came to the understanding that people's capacity to support another person is multifaceted, and they make decisions based on their own capabilities, which is not necessarily indicative of the value of the relationship.

When communicating about cancer and engaging in difficult conversations, expect the unexpected

During my treatment, I was told more than once that cancer can't kill friendship. This is a lovely thought, and one that I would like to think would be generally true. But I came to find that not only in cancer, but also in cases of dramatic accidents and tragic life-altering situations, those on whom you call may, and likely will, tend to fall out of touch pretty quickly. There are circumstances where cancer cannot kill friendship, but they are the exception. Those circumstances have nothing to do with cancer itself, but rather everything to do with the specific bond.

My sister and mother are my best friends. My sister went to the darkest places that cancer took me and stayed alongside me every step of the way. No matter how painful, no matter how difficult it was for her to watch. She stayed with me as I died slowly, and was by my side as I wilted from the horrors of cancer. When it came to the point where I had to face my own mortality, reconciled my soul, and approached the very real and imminent end of my life, she did not shy away from the conversation. Alyce never left me or looked at me any differently than she had when we were young, riding our horses through the hills, racing back, late for dinner, galloping into the sunset.

My sister was traumatized by the idea of losing me to cancer. She would spend every minute of every spare second she had by my side watching Netflix, painting our nails, or gossiping about celebrities on the Internet. And we loved every minute of it.

Even though she was a single mother at the time, as well as studying to get her accounting and CPA license, Alyce made absolutely sure that she would be allowed to spend evenings with me next to my hospital bed. Although she is younger, she has always been a bit protective that way, and I love this about her. Even as a child, she protected our family like no one else I have ever met. She's truly a rock and will go to the ends of the earth (and back) if asked.

In the end, I didn't ask her to go there with me, because she would have without question. But that was not something that I was ever going to ask her to do. It was a war that I did not want her to have to experience alongside me. It was one that I would ultimately face alone.

In the beginning, around January 2012, when I began my chemotherapy, it wasn't entirely evident yet that particular individuals were uncomfortable, or unconsciously positioning themselves away from being involved in my life. I have a vast family between my father's and my mother's relatives. On each side, I have more cousins than I can count and several aunts and uncles. A few years prior to my cancer diagnosis, my grandmother passed away, and there were some residual feelings of anger left over in my once very close extended family. In a very strange way, my cancer forced my family to come together again. It was almost a blessing; it was a life-altering challenge that required so many of us to look beyond the situations of the past and to look forward to finding a solution for what lay ahead of us.

Even before BEACOPP, before scans had shown a recurrence of my cancer, my body was shutting down; my bones ached with a deep pain from the Neupogen shots, which required me to take pain medication, which did nothing for my fatigue aside from exacerbating it. I couldn't stand longer than just a few minutes. I could barely eat anything or keep up with the conversation at the dinner table with family and friends, despite often being the center of the conversation.

In spite of all of this, without fail, there were countless toasts at every dinner party, every family dinner, and every social event to my health, to me. This was not because I was an extraordinary person or had made some substantial contribution to mankind, but rather just that I was sick, I was young, I was bright, I was ambitious, and I was dying.

The day I learned that my cancer had broken through frontline chemotherapy, and I would be on the new higher dose chemotherapy regimen with a much higher toxicity rate, my aunt and uncles had all shown up, and we decided to make a party out of it. It was a Thursday, and they had brought a massive amount of Italian food from this authentic restaurant to the hospital for us all to celebrate. When my Aunt Mary first walked in, I was lying there distraught and near a nervous breakdown in my hospital bed. She exclaimed, "This is the best day ever!" Without having to be sad, I was seriously confused in the beginning. I wondered if she had gotten the wrong news. I thought perhaps she heard I was cured of my cancer. However, that was not the case; she simply had a different reasoning. She viewed the day that we discovered my recurrence as the best day ever because it was the day that we caught my aggressive cancer just in the nick of time. And every Thursday after that, my Aunt Mary and Uncle Steve brought dinner to the hospital room while I was getting BEACOPP. We had wonderful times and excellent dinners, and in all honesty, when the time came for them to leave, it was very difficult for me. Those were good conversations, easy conversations, and I wanted them to go on and on.

✦

At the time that I was diagnosed, many online patient communities had not yet been launched and were still in beta. These online patient networks provide members access to medical resources, experts, data, and studies, as well as give patients and survivors opportunities to connect with one other. This can be access to more information than local support groups provide.

I have watched online communities as they have developed over the past few years, and I can personally attest to the benefits good ones can provide. These forums are an invaluable resource for any patient who is looking to become an active participant in their healthcare, and to take on a larger role in the management of their health. To be an active patient, it is absolutely essential that you have access to the best information and knowledge sources available. Being a member of these knowledge-sharing communities gives you the ability to contact medical experts and to receive additional counseling resources. Also, it gives you the opportunity to connect with other cancer patients and survivors.

Good groups are not just made of casual observers, but of members who take a sincere and strong interest in patients and what their struggles are. For anyone seeking support through and after cancer treatment, a knowledgeable group can provide one of the strongest and caring support networks that I have ever come across.

I strongly encourage any person considering joining an online community to do so. This is one of the most vital resources that I use. I sincerely regret not finding this knowledge and support resource when I was first diagnosed, and I hope you take full advantage of everything these support groups have to offer.

These communities are also important because doctors will be able to gain from them. When we are considering the type of benefits that the physician and clinical practitioners can gain from a patient community it is important to respect the culture and the amount of dedication, work, and long hours that each physician has put in to become an expert in his or her field. Doctor bashing helps no one.

This respect revolves around the concept that doctors have earned their position as experts and this alone demands respect. However, the truth is that few practitioners and clinicians have directly experienced the illnesses they treat; therefore a doctor needs his or her patient's experience in order to have a comprehensive perspective on the matter.

There are aspects of treatment and illness that the medical community learns from patients and caregivers—not through research studies and lab tests alone—that would greatly benefit the overall expertise of practitioners and clinicians. If a doctor were open to the idea of including a patient's experience into the way they manage health care, he or she would become a more well-rounded clinician.

# CHAPTER ELEVEN

# THE WAR ON CANCER AND THE BATTLE OF THE RIBBONS

*Cancer wasn't some opponent I could defeat; it was a disease. It was within my own body. No matter how angry I got or how hard I tried, I couldn't kill my opponent, not without also killing myself.*

✦

Once I got cancer, I learned the language pretty quickly. I had no choice.

"If anyone can beat cancer, you can!"

"Don't worry, I have faith in you that you will beat this!"

I started noticing the loaded language. People didn't *have* cancer; they were at war with it.

"He/she/I lost the battle with cancer."

"He/she/I won the war with cancer."

The language surrounding the issue of cancer is unusual and can be a taboo topic that plays a central role in modern cancer culture. Oftentimes when a patient enters remission or what is currently referred to as "No Evidence of Disease" (NED), the patient is said to have "won their battle" with cancer. Alternatively, if the patient has died, they are often referred to as having "lost their battle" with cancer.

The use of heavily militarized and combative terminology used within today's modern cancer culture is, in my experience, intriguing, inapplicable, and overdramatic. The language of battle implies that there is a winner and that there is a loser. However, it also implies that there is an element of effort that the patient must put forth in order to "win."

Many times during my "battle" with cancer, I was told, "You are the strongest person I know!" This usually came in concert with the inevitable,

"If anyone can beat this, you can!" This created a fear of failure like if I tried just hard enough, I could win and cancer would lose. It does not work this way. The implication that the patient's pure strength and will to survive will determine the outcome is misguided, especially among terminal cancer patients.

In a recent documentary called *Pink Ribbons Inc.*, a stage IV cancer support group for women debated this topic and shared how the language of cancer made them feel. It made them feel that they had failed, that they were not enough. Ultimately, the patients in this group looked back at what they could have done differently and often blamed themselves. They carried a certain amount of guilt regarding their condition. However, these women mainly resented the way the language of cancer had lowered their self-worth. I understood their feelings. Cancer wasn't some opponent I could defeat; it was a disease. It was within my own body. No matter how angry I got or how hard I tried, I couldn't kill my opponent, not without also killing myself.

I can understand how for caregivers like my mother, they feel that they are battling cancer and are in some sort of war for the high ground. I can understand how caregivers and our loved ones often feel this way because, to them, cancer is an external force that they are constantly having to adjust and rearrange their lives around.

For those of us who received treatment of the slash, burn, and poison variety, no matter where we were with our "war" against cancer, it should've been easy to spot the losers. Losers disappeared from infusion mid-treatment; they went into the hospital and didn't come out; they were relegated to hospice. We noticed their absence but didn't keep score. If they were the losers, we would've seen the winners victorious. But the cancer died along with them. When someone dies from cancer, nobody wins.

Cancer patients are often faced with what is commonly referred to as the "cancer culture." Filled with colorful ribbons and an overabundance of optimism, cancer patients will often try to appease doctors, family members, friends, and caregivers by sharing in this optimistic approach. While this in itself may not be harmful to the patient, this desire to conform can lead to the crowding out of the patient's real emotions, making it difficult for the patient to discuss difficult topics such as mortality, fear of recurrence, and other concerns. Without the ability to honestly express these feelings, the patient may turn inward and begin to isolate or even resent those with this optimistic outlook. This, as a result, will often emotionally separate the patient from the people who are there in a supportive role and as caregivers.

There are more than twenty-five types of cancer ribbons. That's more colors than the standard Crayola crayon box. Aside from selling cancer ribbons, vendors sell cancer watches, jewelry, Bibles, stickers, clothing, and even dog accessories. Much of it is pink and for breast cancer. There were times when people would leave me gifts at the hospital, which was very sweet. However, every time they left me a gift it was pink galore. My ribbon color was violet. So people tend to ignore any cancer ribbon that isn't pink. People who have a black cancer ribbon have been rebranding themselves with the slogan "black is the new pink."

I was talking to a director at University of Texas Southwestern who happened to be a breast cancer survivor. The breast ward there had ribbons, balloons, flowers—it looked more like a maternity ward than a cancer unit. It was definitely an upgrade from where the rest of us cancer patients got treated. I noticed they even had bottles of water, where the rest of us, the sickest patients, had to drink tap water. I asked the director why they had water bottles, flowers, decorations—they even had an exclusive breast cancer library. She explained that the breast cancer unit had more funding because they had more survivors. People don't want to donate to people who are just going to die. They wouldn't even allow us other patients to touch any of the library books or have a bottle of water.

That's the battle of the ribbons. The pink cancer culture vs. the rest of us ribbons.

✦

In order for a cancer treatment to have been successful, it is commonly believed that it will put the patient into remission. This is not always the case. For those of us who have been diagnosed with late stage or terminal cancer, this may not even be a card that's on the table.

Cancer as a battle, a war, an evil, means that even when the patient may have been given multiple years of prolonged life that was meaningful and enjoyable, should they pass away from a cancer-related cause, it is very common to read an obituary that begins with some version of the following: "John Smith lost his battle with cancer on Tuesday evening after years of struggle."

It alarms me that despite being gifted with the longevity of a life that otherwise would not have been afforded, if you have cancer and you die, our culture will say you lost your battle.

In losing this war with cancer, and in rather drastic terms, using a militaristic language used by generals in combat, it implies that the patient had some amount of control over whether or not the battle or a war was to be won or lost. We begin to hear comments from those around us by friends and family to the tune of, "You can beat this. You're a fighter!" In a nutshell, the amount of courage or sheer willpower to survive becomes what is expected of us. Not fighting hard enough becomes an affront to those relentlessly cheering us on.

I had the characteristics, I suppose, that make up a cancer winner. I was strong-willed, tenacious, and aggressive when it came to achieving my goals. Surely, if anyone could beat this cancer scourge ... But wearing that mantle into battle was not a burden or responsibility I wanted to have placed on my shoulders. Eventually, I will almost undoubtedly die of cancer or a cancer-related issue, but I will die well. No battle ribbons, please, I can't keep up with all the colors.

Yes. It will be a cold day in hell when any person who attends my funeral, no matter how many years from now, stands up and says publicly anything like, "Sarah Kugler Powers lost her battle with cancer this past Tuesday. She fought courageously for eighty years before she finally lost her war." A cold day in hell.

It is time to redefine how we see failure and what we see as a success when it comes to cancer. I am no loser. And I refuse to see cancer as ever being a winner.

CHAPTER TWELVE

# SUPPORT SYSTEMS AND CAREGIVERS

*"A seriously ill child tests the strength of every individual and every relationship. Some endure, even thrive, while others weaken or even shatter. There is no way to prepare for the challenge, because a family's journey to the valley of the shadow of death almost always comes on without warning."~Alan Dershowitz*

✦

A support system is crucial to pretty much any endeavor in life, but never so important as during cancer treatment. Be it family, friends, or a support group, no one does it alone. Or at least, they shouldn't.

Ideally a patient will have a primary caregiver—a primary support person to be the hub of all that needs to be done during treatment. The caregiver will not only physically assist the patient when needed, but will provide emotional and psychological support as well. He or she will make sure the wheels of treatment keep turning—appointments met, paperwork filed, medications filled. A primary caregiver can (and should) be part of a larger support network, but he or she is the one who helps the patient with the day-in day-out minutiae of living through cancer treatment.

If a patient does not identify either a support system or caregiver, it is likely that the patient will have a greater struggle with cancer diagnosis and treatment. No one should go it alone.

Most major hospitals, including Stanford University Medical Center, provide resources for support groups and classes for caregivers so that they have people to turn to themselves when the load gets too heavy to carry alone. Burnout is common for caregivers, as is illness. They work so hard at taking care of the patient that they forget to take care of themselves. Patients need to stay engaged and keep an eye on their caregivers whenever possible to make sure they don't lose themselves in the patient's illness.

When two people enter into a caregiver and patient relationship, it is vital to have a frank discussion about what the relationship will look like. Setting up personal boundaries in advance can help to mitigate disagreements in the future. Although not all situations are predictable, it might be useful for the two parties to talk through some hypothetical situations to ensure they're on the same page.

My mother is my primary caregiver. She stepped into that role without my having to ask and before I even knew I was going to need her. My cancer was so advanced and it progressed so quickly, we didn't have time to discuss the parameters of our relationship, nor did we even have the language to do so. In many ways, we both regressed to the roles we'd played when I was a child. Sometimes this worked fine; sometimes I fought to re-establish my agency as an adult. But I was always thankful to have her with me during every step of treatment.

As the child of my caregiver and also the patient, my relationship with my mother as primary caregiver was often painful and challenging for both of us. Following my first recurrence, which made BEACOPP necessary and sent me down the path to a bone marrow transplant, when things were at their worst, every day as I lay in my hospital bed with my mom by my side, I was comforted. But I could also see the amount of pain that my illness was causing her. The thought of losing her child to cancer at such a young age was something that she could never discuss, and to date that is a conversation we have never had.

My mother always tried to remain optimistic in hopes of keeping my spirits up, while she suffered in silence, crying herself to sleep at night and attempting to cope with, and process her own terror and fears privately. In her way, she felt that if she remained a constant source of encouragement and hope that her relentless positivity would be my anchor in the storm, unwavering and resilient. Without fail, there was never a day that I did not have her by my side doing all she could, praying that it just might be enough to save my life.

Nothing pains me more than knowing that my mother was suffering horribly and alone, all while attempting to create an environment that was positive, loving, and upbeat for me, twenty-four hours a day, seven days a week. At one point I did try to discuss this with her, but she completely shut down and remained resolute and determined to ensure that at all times she remained strong for the both of us. I know that without her dedication and tough love, I would not be alive today.

On the other hand, this meant that I processed my own fears about death, as well as my final preparations, alone. When I had finally completed everything I needed to leave things in order after my passing, I reached a very calm peaceful place where I had accepted my failures, owned my successes, and let go of any anger and ill will that I was holding onto. I was sincerely ready to go. But I never told my mother.

The morning that I thought was my last was at the Stanford cancer center where my team of oncologists was prepping me for my bone marrow transplant. I had become extremely ill. I was no longer able to walk; I was no longer able to eat or drink, and just about the only thing I could do was listen to my audiobooks and the podcasts my law professors from the University of Connecticut would upload.

The previous night had been one of the most difficult of my entire life. I'd heard of coming-to-Jesus moments and dark nights of the soul, but now I understood just what those terms meant.

By morning, I had nothing left to draw upon. I had exhausted any will I had to survive, any hope, and all physical and mental strength. At about six o'clock that morning, I promised myself that I would let myself pass that day, and stop resisting the inevitable, as long as I could survive long enough to see my mother. I had two hours to go. I couldn't even open my eyes, let alone speak or grieve. I felt trapped in this dying body as my mind raced. I knew that my mother would come through those doors at 8:00 am, with that smile on her face and peppy tone in her voice, and I wanted to see that one more time and to hold her hand one more time. I never anticipated I would live longer than about an hour after she finally arrived.

Trying to keep my mind awake for those two hours turned out to be completely impossible. I'm not sure what time I fell asleep, despite my best efforts, but when I woke up it was after my mother had arrived. I opened my eyes to look over at my mom, and there she was in the chair next to my bed fast asleep, her body slumped over in complete exhaustion. She looked weak, as if she had aged fifteen years, and my heart just broke. I hadn't seen her sleep since I had been diagnosed, and I watched her for as long as I could before the next dose of morphine kicked in. Just before I went back into my morphine-induced doze, I just prayed for strength to keep going despite my entire being screaming to be let go. I just could not leave her. I may have been ready, but she was not.

If you are a caregiver, what I hope you take away from this chapter is that even when we are deathly ill, in states induced with heavy pain, anxiety, and sleep medications, we see you. Whether we are suffering in silence, or, as in my case, holding a filibuster every time I had an ache or pain, we see what you do for us. We see the toll that it takes on you to care for us. We see the pain and the challenges, as well as the life changes that you've had to make to care for us. Too many caregivers have told me that they have no right to ever complain or discuss feelings of depression, fear, or anxiety or anything else that they think might create a negative environment for the patient, and so they do exactly what my mother did and suffer in private, but we see that too.

Speaking from my personal experience, I can say that it pains us to see you suffer in silence. If I could go back and change one thing about the relationship between my mother and me in terms of her being my primary caregiver, I would tell her that it is OK for her to feel these types of emotions, and that I needed her to be honest with me about how she was coping with and managing everything she had to take on. There was a lot of pain in those hospital rooms, even when it was with just the two of us, and in hindsight, I believe that if we could have been more open and honest about how we were managing, it would have eased the burdens and challenges that we took on together over those years.

✦

All patients and their partners will feel stress about their changing relationship. Dealing with the numerous changes can be difficult. However,
some couples find their bond becomes stronger during this drastically
difficult time.

To reduce the stress, remind yourself that everyone handles things
differently, and you and your spouse aren't doing anything wrong. Any
effort made toward solutions is a good thing. Try to be open with each
other about the stress and what is causing it for each of you. Try and remove
pressure from your partner's life. For example, if a mess in the house stresses
your spouse, try and clean up. Share with each other about how you are
both coping, and come up with additional coping strategies together. Try
to be grateful for one another and the bond that you have. Make time to
focus on things besides cancer such as going on a romantic date or having
a movie night at home. Take a walk together or cook a healthy meal for
each other. Stay dialed in and considerate. If ever there were a time to put
the Golden Rule at the forefront of your relationship, this is it. Treat each
other as you want to be treated.

While some dynamics and advice are the same no matter the relationship
between patient and caregiver, couples have a challenge others don't. Sex.

Your partner may feel different about your sex life during treatment
than you do. This could be for several reasons. Your partner may not feel
as attractive under the effects of cancer. Treatment may be affecting your
partner's ability to perform, or your partner is physically tired or depressed.
In spite of these issues, you can try to remain close and intimate. Talk about
being close, talk about your sex life. Talk about your hopes for your future
without judging each other. Make sure you set time aside for just you and
your partner to talk. Talk to a counselor or support group. Talk.

Being sick can be especially difficult for young people diagnosed with
cancer. They are likely the youngest people in the infusion rooms and thus
feel isolated from other patients. Additionally, young cancer patients tend
to make up a smaller demographic. This often causes feelings of separation
from their peer group. Their close friends often have no context for what
they're going through, and may be insensitive to the cancer patient's feelings
or what they're going through. The patient will likely experience body

image issues, changes in intimacy and sex, and changes in fertility. This will serve to both diminish the patient's self-esteem and put a strain on romantic relationships.

Fertility issues also play a complicated role in the psychological well-being of young patients. Many patients find their fertility is negatively impacted by cancer treatment during their prime childbearing years. This may cause feelings of depression among young patients who were planning on having children. Other patients may feel resentment toward their peers who seem to be "popping out babies" left and right. These issues just serve to further drive a wedge between the young cancer patient and his or her loved ones.

As loved ones of these cancer patients, what can anyone do to show friendship and support during this trying period? First, it is essential that supporters offer help but make it specific. Just offering to "help" puts the burden of coming up with something for the supporter to do on the patient, and the patient probably won't end up asking. Offering to come over and help clean the house or cook a meal is more specific and easier for the patient to accept. (One thing to note about cooking for or bringing food for cancer patients is due to their treatment, they often experience an extreme change in taste. So the friend who used to love banana cream pie may despise it now. Make sure to double check with your friend on changing tastes. Instead of cooking a meal, try stocking the pantry with all of your friend's new favorite foods.) Offer to take kids to school or walk the dog. Pets and children need care during this time and the patient may not be able to handle it all.

When it comes to asking for or even receiving help, many women are resistant. They're independent and strong and don't want assistance. Being part of a support network means reminding the patient that nobody is an island and explaining she may get something out of being helped. At the very least, she needs to know that offers of help from others are not only for her, but they're also comforting for the people offering. Not allowing people to help is hurtful to them. Hopefully, she will allow people to support her.

Another way to do something positive for a friend with cancer is to read that person's cancer web page and blog or help create a cancer web page or blog. Creating these sites allows patients to update multiple people at one time without having to call each person individually. Also, having a blog allows the freedom to write about feelings. Patients can also use their web page to ask for the kind of help they truly need.

Yet another important aspect of supporting a friend with cancer is listening. If a patient wants to talk about his or her cancer, it is important that supporters not tell the patient how to feel about the situation. No one outside the medical team should be giving advice unless the patient asks for it. Just listen.

Cancer treatment is hectic. Supporters can offer to drive the patient to appointments or to pick up prescriptions. They can be a second set of ears and eyes in appointments by taking notes and listening to everything the doctor says. A supporter can help give a patient confidence when it comes to being his or her own advocate.

Naturally, a supporter is usually welcome to spoil the patient rotten with gifts, treats, and surprises. Anything to get the patient's mind off of cancer. Supporters can send her cards and funny presents. They can spend time with the patient doing what he or she wants to do or even nothing at all. However, it is important to remember the patient is sick. He or she may have to cancel plans at the last minute, or may not return a phone call. A supporter needs to be ready to forgive these things.

Lastly, supporters need to remember that cancer is a long journey. Supporters don't disappear on their friends. Even recovery is rough; patients need support through that too. Supporters stick it out through the fun times (and those do exist) and the tough times. That's what makes their presence support.

✦

You may not think of yourself as a caregiver because you're doing something "natural" and taking care of someone you love. But if you're helping a loved one through cancer treatment, then you are indeed a caregiver. As a caregiver, it's normal to listen to the patient's feelings and put your feelings to the wayside. However, putting your needs to the side for too long is not healthy for you and it may hinder your ability to care for others.

The role of caregiver may be a new, and it's OK to feel stressed. Many caregivers join support groups to help them get through this difficult period. Being in a support group helps the caregiver to communicate more efficiently with the patient and helps them be able to vocalize things they weren't able to before by giving them tools for patient communication.

Aside from stress, there are other feelings caregivers may experience. They may feel guilty, which is exceedingly common. They may feel like they aren't helping enough. Or they may feel guilty that they are healthy, and the person they care about is sick. They may even feel angry. It is not uncommon for a caregiver to be angry with a patient for a whole variety of reasons (from not picking up their socks to refusing to take medications) and not know how to handle it.

Caregivers may be overcome with grief. They may grieve for their former life before they were so needed. They may grieve the loss of a loved one's health. They must let themselves grieve these things and air these emotions. It's OK to feel sad. But if the sadness lasts more than two weeks they may have depression and might want to seek medical care. Their feelings are natural, and they are doing all they can do at this point in their life. Patients need to remember not to take the caregiver's feelings personally (just as the caregiver needs to not take it personally when the patient is going through all the same emotions).

Although caregivers may feel like their needs are the last thing they should be worrying about, it's important for them to take time for themselves. Sometimes they need to just take a break. Ask close friends or family members to pitch in so they can rest. It may feel awkward, but you'll be surprised at how many people are willing help out during this time. Encourage caregivers to spend time with friends, family, and pets. Have them take the dog for a walk or email a close friend. Ask them to do something nice for themselves, such as work on a hobby or go to a movie with a friend. Remind them (nicely) to take care of their body. Make sure they are getting enough exercise, getting enough rest, and eating healthy foods. Lastly, encourage them to join a caregiver support group where they can talk about their feelings with other people who are experiencing the same things they are and can give advice. It helps to know they're not alone.

✦

Cancer in the workplace elicits a host of questions for the newly diagnosed. The first is whether they will be able to be successful in their role while in cancer treatment and during recovery. The second is more technical as the patient must become thoroughly acquainted with the organization's benefits and insurance programs. The third question, and maybe the most delicate in the day-to-day life of a patient, is how will they be viewed in the workplace when the proverbial cat is out of the bag.

Let's face it: most if not all of us want to be seen as an indispensable part of any work team, always at the ready should the need arise. A cancer diagnosis physically changes this. Often, patients fear that decreasing their hours, taking time off for appointments and treatment, or simply asking for help will be seen as falling behind. Or worse, a paternalistic boss might think that the patient's workload should in some way be lessened. It is important in dealing with workplace issues that patients become aware of federal and state labor laws, benefit programs, and insurances that may be provided by either the government or their employer. The specifics will often depend on the type of employer, the size of the organization, and other various factors.

I was diagnosed with stage IV cancer at the age of twenty-four, and I can attest to the hesitation for young cancer patients to reach out to others for support or to really discuss openly their cancer treatment or really anything to do with their personal cancer experience in general. I know what it feels like to be the youngest person in the chemotherapy room. And when I say youngest, I mean I've got most of these people by a good forty years.

Cancer patients at different ages think about different things. A six-ty-five year old is not thinking of job security or potential fertility issues. Sixty-five year olds, while not necessarily being OK with the thought of their own mortality, might not necessarily be thinking about all that lies ahead. Without an implicit motive, being the baby in the room encourages feelings of, sometimes, gross abnormality.

As a young adult, I was expected to fit in with my peers and my colleagues both at work and at play. This made it difficult because so often the secondary pubescence of becoming a stable and productive human being reveals just as many growing pains as the initial change a decade prior. Now that cancer was part of this metamorphosis, I inherited a new inability to cope with some of the most basic and simple tasks of everyday life. It paved an unwanted road leading to a mutual alienation between everyone involved: friends, co-workers, and me.

Cancer changes things. It changes people. It changes the way some people treated me. This is not their failure or evidence of poor character, but how they related to me as a young cancer patient on an experiential level. Our lives were ultimately so different it became hard to find a comfortable common ground.

Once someone discovered I was sick, the standard "My aunt's cousin's ex-teacher's brother's lover's former roommate's gardener's great grandfather had cancer" came up. I could have really turned up the heat by asking, "Did they live?" I knew, though, that their intention was simply to relate to an almost un-relatable situation.

And how, really, should I have responded to something like that? "Cancer? That's awful." And if I say that, I'm saying that it's awful that I have it, too. In fact, I might as well have taken a sharpie and written on my forehead, "I have a handicap and it's called cancer!" It means I am, at least at present, different. It means I'm special in a bad way. It means I'm less of a peer.

It means I'm sick.

The interesting part is that it brought out the best and worst in people at the same time. The hugs got a little bit longer and voices got a little (or a lot) gentler. However, if I sneezed, Steven King himself might as well have entered the room saying, "Sarah, it's time."

But I couldn't really tell anyone this at the time because I didn't understand any of it. If there is any learned or ingrained knowledge in our culture of the extent that cancer impacts a life, young adults can take that number and slash it by three-fourths. That's how much I did not know.

What I did know became second nature by the sheer repetition of the conversations. It was lather, rinse, and repeat answers to the same questions.

*Yes, it is stage IV.*

*No there is no stage V.*

*Yes, this is a wig.*

*I can neither confirm nor deny whether I inhaled, which is a mute point because I have a state-issued card anyway.*

*No, you cannot borrow it.*

Kid gloves did not begin to describe my interactions. Think more like baby mittens, the kind used to keep newborns from scratching themselves with those ten little razor blades at the end of their phalanges. My colleagues did not speak to me the way they had B.C. (before cancer). It was rather disturbing to watch people working very hard to not upset me or hurt my feelings. And in a really odd twist of fate, latitude afforded me had more to do with my follicles than with anything else. I was given extra time on projects, and the standards were a bit more flexible for me the balder I became.

Then I lost my eyebrows. And they lost their minds.

My Uncle Fester stunt-double hobby birthed an unnecessary episode of "Workplace Limbo." I always thought the point of limbo was, "How low can you go?" And everyone not named Sarah Kugler Powers was playing against each other competitively and as equals. But when the bald girl wanted a turn, the stick magically found itself with just a bit... or a foot... of leeway that I never asked for, nor wanted. It made it impossible for me to truly compete with my colleagues and peers, which was one of the more enjoyable aspects of my job. It was an unwritten rule that I would no longer have to bend over backwards in order to compete in the workplace.

Standards lowered. Stick raised. God, I hate pity.

# CHAPTER THIRTEEN

# ANOTHER POINT OF VIEW: ALAN DERSHOWITZ ON BEING PARENT AND CAREGIVER

Alan Dershowitz is one of the greatest legal minds of the modern era, but the wealth of wisdom and his contributions to society are vast and extend far beyond the law. I look up to Alan as a great and wise mind, as a scholar, a legal practitioner, and also as a friend and mentor. Through his work, and writings Alan has become one of the largest influences in my life, and I have been very blessed to have learned valuable life lessons during the time we have known each other. I hope you enjoy the following contribution from Alan Dershowitz, who shares with you his experience.

*By the early 1970s, I had become well established as a young academic, as a budding First Amendment lawyer, and as a father. Life was good. Suddenly everything changed. My older son, Elon, fell while playing hockey, hit his head on the ice, and was taken, unconscious, to St. Elizabeth's Hospital. Nobody was sure whether he had fainted before he hit his head or whether the impact with the ice had caused his unconsciousness. The initial diagnosis was adolescent epilepsy, which was treated pharmaceutically.*

*In the summer of 1971, the family traveled by car to Palo Alto, California, where I was to take up residency for a year at the Center for Advanced Study in Behavioral Sciences. My project was to complete a long, scholarly book titled Predictive Justice: Toward a Jurisprudence of Harm Prevention. It was an ambitious project for a thirty-three year- old academic, but I felt up to the task of formulating a new legal framework for what I saw as the emerging "preventive state."*

*The center, located adjacent to the Stanford University Campus, was a unique institution. It would invite approximately forty scholars from around the world, each from different disciplines that touched on behavioral sciences. I was the only law professor that year, among a group that included the philosopher Robert Nozick, the political theorist Michael Walzer, the linguists Robin and George Lako, the psychologists Philip Zimbardo and Amos Tversky, the sociologist Nathan Glazer, the psychiatrist Albert Stunkard, the Romanian economist Michael Cernea, and the psychoanalyst Bruno Bettelheim.*

*We were each assigned a small cabin in which to write our own books, but we were expected to join the others for luncheon talks and seminar presentations. Collaborations were encouraged, and many fine books emerged from the serene hills of Palo Alto. Mine, however, was not among them. In early December, after I had completed my historical research and writing, my son Elon was diagnosed with a malignant brain tumor--a diagnosis missed by the Boston doctors in the days before CT scans.*

*The first person to suggest the dreaded diagnosis was Bruno Bettelheim, who worked in the adjoining cabin and invited me for "high tea," which his Viennese-born wife would bring him every afternoon. Although Bruno was not a physician--indeed he had never been able to complete college because of the emergence of Nazism in Germany and Austria-- he had studied with Sigmund Freud and was regarded as one of the most distinguished, though controversial, psychoanalytic thinkers in the world.*

*When I told him about my son's recurring headaches and seizures, his first comment was "Remember George Gershwin?" I was a great fan of Gershwin's music, and family lore suggested we might even be related, since his original name was Gershowitz, and the Gs, Ds, and Hs sometimes got mixed up at Ellis Island. But I didn't know what Bruno was referring to. He explained: "Gershwin had headaches for years and underwent lengthy psychoanalysis by analysts who believed that every pain was caused by early childhood experiences, and could be treated by the talking cure. Eventually, it was discovered, he had a brain tumor from which he died at age thirty-eight."*

*Following this morbid conversation, I took Elon to Stanford Hospital, where a brain scan disclosed a tumor. We rushed him to Boston's Children's Hospital, where a remarkable neurosurgeon, John Shilito, removed it. We then returned to Stanford, where another remarkable doctor, Henry Kaplan, performed radiation therapy over several months.*

*I did not have enough money to afford this extraordinary medical care, and Judge David Bazelon--who was Elon's godfather--loaned me what I needed. He also loaned me money to invest in a real estate venture with a friend of his in Washington, Charles E. Smith. The return on that venture allowed me to pay off my loan to Bazelon over several years, but I vowed never again to require help from others to take care of my family's medical needs. From then on, I began to charge clients who could afford my legal services. Within a few years, I had saved enough to be able to pay for any medical or other family emergency.*

*When I returned to the center at Stanford, nothing was the same. I couldn't concentrate on my book. My marriage, which had been suffering for several years even before our trip to California, was now in deep trouble. All I could think about and work on was my son's condition. The clock was always ticking. The doctors told me that if he made it past a year, the odds of his survival would go up, and if he made it past two years, they would go up even more. These years went by very slowly, with several scares but thankfully no recurrence.*

*During this time I spent hours in the medical library, learning all I could about Elon's condition. The doctors were encouraging but the research was not. (Research has no bedside manner!) Although I did not turn to religion as a source of solace, I did read and reread the book of Job, a remarkable story about how human beings confront tragedy. When God decided to test Job's faith, his first action was to afflict his children. The author of Job understood, as anyone who has experienced the serious*

*illness of a child understands, that there is no greater test a parent con-
fronts than when a child faces death.*

*Everything changes. Life is put on hold. Samuel Johnson once observed
that nothing focuses the mind quite as clearly as an appointment with the
hangman. Johnson obviously didn't have a child with cancer. Nothing can
make a parent focus more single-mindedly on any issue than a child with
a life-threatening illness and the steps that must be taken to maximize
the chances of survival, both physical and psychological.*

*I have discussed this issue with friends who have lived through life-threat-
ening illnesses suffered by their children. Some, like me, try to become
super-scientists, reading everything they can get their hands on, conferring
with every expert they can reach, and micromanaging every medical
decision. Others leave these matters to the doctors and devote themselves to
showering their child with love and support. Still others found it difficult
to engage either scientifically or emotionally. Every parent is different, as
are the needs of every child. Illness among children does not come with a
one-size-fits-all instruction manual. The first priority, of course, is the life
of the child, but not far behind is the psychological welfare, both short- and
long-term, of the child who survives the illness.*

*One common reaction among parents of seriously ill children who have
made it through the initial treatment phase is to try to bury the difficult
memories by not thinking or talking about the traumatic past. With cancer
survivors this is especially problematic, since the threat of recurrence is
ever present, and past may become prologue. Healthy vigilance must be
balanced against unhealthy obsession with every possible symptom. The
struggle never ends. The scars, though sometimes invisible, remain.*

*A seriously ill child tests the strength of every individual and every
relationship. Some endure, even thrive, while others weaken or even
shatter. There is no way to prepare for the challenge, because a family's
journey to the valley of the shadow of death almost always comes on
without warning.*

There are several stages a parent goes through during and following the diagnosis. The first involves immediate panic, overwhelming frustration, and a sense of helplessness. This may be followed by intense involvement in the treatment process. Then there is the treatment itself--often surgery followed by radiation and chemotherapy. Finally, there is waiting--a year, five years, ten years--before one can be relatively confident that the treatment has worked. During this waiting period, it becomes difficult to concentrate on anything else, as your child seems cured, but you know there is the lingering fear of recurrence. I could not focus on long-term projects. I needed short deadlines that did not allow my mind to wander.

But wander it did, to my child's future, to whether I was subtly treating him differently because of his encounter with illness, to every minor symptom that might signal a recurrence. Elon is the hero in this saga. The doctors told him that the surgery might affect his manual dexterity. His hobby was close-up magic, which requires extraordinary dexterity.

He was determined to prove the doctors wrong, so he worked endlessly on his moves. Before the surgery, he had a magic act that he performed to friends and some Stanford fraternities. He had billed himself "Elon the Pretty Good." Following the surgery he quickly became, at least to me, "Elon the Great," performing at Boston Celtics Christmas parties, Patrick Kennedy's birthday party, and at the Legal Sea Foods Restaurant. More importantly, he performed for kids with brain tumors and other neurological problems at hospitals and radiation centers, even when he himself was undergoing radiation therapy.

It was a difficult time for all of us, but Elon's determination lifted our spirits. Nor did Elon's friends (and their parents) make it easier on Elon. His closest friend in California was told by his parents to keep his distance from Elon. When I raised the issue with them, they said they did not want their son to become too close to a boy who might die. Schoolmates taunted Elon about his wig and called him "tumor boy." But Elon persisted, even playing football within a year of the surgery.

# CHAPTER FOURTEEN

# BLAME AND HOPE

*Cancer will beat your hopes into submission, and it will take away so much from your life and those you love. But you can refill, and you can rebuild, and you can regenerate your hope for a life that may be even more profound than your original desires.*

✦

O ne of the first questions that comes to mind, and can dominate any patient's thoughts after receiving a cancer diagnosis, is why me? The question is simple. The clarity of an answer lies somewhere between wet mud and a lump of coal.

If a patient has struggled with the *why me* question, he or she needs to consider the type of cancer. Is the cancer one that has a known link to a specific type of behavior, such as smoking? If so, it's not a stretch for patients to feel like personal behavior is the root cause of the disease. However, if a causal link is not present, often a patient will struggle to find a reason for his or her cancer, turning to issues such as nutrition, exercise, or environmental factors.

Self-blame is one of the most insidious natures of this beast. We tend to look for a way to blame ourselves, when sometimes, shit just happens.

I never asked *why me*. I asked *why them*? This is one of the greatest moral and deepest failings that I struggle with in my character. My lifelong faith in God remained as solid as it ever was, so I never thought to question my getting sick. In a way, I saw my relationship with God as ordained, and felt certain my cancer was not without reason. I somehow knew that things would always be OK, or at the very least divinely planned, so I could accept what I had been dealt in life. I never once let cancer impact my faith in my own destiny. Others, however…

What did they do to deserve it?

And then I looked in the mirror, and I saw myself, who survived for no scientific reason or logical understanding. Medically, I should not be here.

And it was not asked as a personal slight to them; I wasn't thinking, "They must have done something to bring it on themselves." Sadly, the truth is far more personally shameful. I asked, *why them* in moments of great anger and pain for the beautiful and cherished lives lost to cancer that I have seen all too often. Why were these people survivors and not people who I personally felt contributed more with their lives. Why did good people die while bad people lived? And which was I?

During some of my lowest points, I cringed at these great losses or when I was around other survivors, asking with anger and challenge, "God, why them? Why them?" What had gotten into me? Was I taunting God? Did my own faith anger me?

At times I could hardly tolerate any type of support group. It felt like the gravity of the lives that were lost rested squarely on the shoulders of my soul. It was so unbelievable that such forces of life and sources of light in the world had been snuffed out. All that remained were others like me, those left to pick up the shattered pieces of our purpose. I'm not sure anyone could even begin to understand the disproportionate value that had been lost. In the balance of nature, I wondered if anything had even been gained. The tallies would forever be unfair.

Since my diagnosis, I have dedicated my life to this work, and will continue to do so until my dying breath. If the effort is going to save just one beautiful and strong life force, then everything I have done and have suffered through has been worth every second of my fate. I ask *why them* a lot. It's motivation. I ask in honor of those who have departed, and I ask for those who have endured beyond all medical odds.

And *them* includes so many people. *Them* includes loved ones. *Them* includes those in the throes of the struggle. *Them* might just include you.

✦

When I think of hope, I am inundated with questions. How do we even begin to define the concept of hope? In the context of cancer, what does hope look like, and is it based solely in the eye of the beholder? Is it possible for each of us to hope in ways that are completely foreign to one another?

And what happens when we transform the power of hope from a tangible idea with real possibilities, to one of delusional fantasy, almost entirely depending upon faith in something or some being; does that make hope potentially dangerous? Can false hope do more harm than good?

Is it possible to defer hope? If a late-stage diagnosis or a series of set-backs shatters it across the landscape of the journey, is it possible to simply mute it in the attempt to manage our expectations and our emotions to match a particular situation or circumstance? Or do we defer hope so that we willingly give it up so that it cannot be taken from us by something so cruel as cancer?

Is it easier for us to give up hope, to defer, to rationalize it into another form such as faith, which does not require us to place ourselves so deeply and solely within a particular hope? In other words, when we do not achieve the results we are looking for, are there reasons behind the suffering or do bad things simply happen?

Personally, I think cancer can shatter hope, and I have seen cancer do away with it entirely. And it doesn't take long for the transformation to happen. A relapse, a tumor that won't shrink, or dipping your toe into the sea of depression is all it takes.

We let go of hope. We delay hope. We misplace hope. And then if we can't quite find where we put it, we trade hope for faith. Faith allows us to bridge the gaps, to put stock in something of which we have no control if and when we finally get to that spot. To lose hope and to begin to run on faith is not as difficult of a transition as you might think, but the danger occurs when faith no longer has any basis in hope. The two tend to comingle quite symbiotically, but faith divorced from hope is one of the darkest and most tormenting conditions of man.

I cannot transform how you see your concept of hope. With cancer, it will be challenged in so many seen and unseen ways. Cancer attacks everything indiscriminately, and a never-ending avalanche of difficulties can turn holding on to hope into an exercise in futility.

However, I have learned that while cancer can and will shatter hopes and dreams in every way imaginable, hope has the power to transform, to evolve, and to overcome cancer, even if the eventual outcome is ultimately death.

When I was first diagnosed, I hoped for a cure, as did my family. I not only hoped for a life that would be free of cancer and its malicious effects but also relied on this hope in such a serious and fervent way that I framed my entire life around it.

For so many reasons and in so many ways, my hope was stripped, torn and burned by cancer. Any vision I had of leading a relatively normal life or having the life that I had always perceived as a guarantee, was destroyed. I had nothing of that life now, and I had no hope for it returning.

However, I learned to hope again when I learned to hope for a different life. I began to hope for a life that would bring great meaning and kindness and good to the world. I had hope that my life, which had now irreversibly changed, would become a mosaic from the fragmented pieces of my old dreams, a mosaic in which others could see their own reflection, and in so doing, learn a great deal about themselves and their experience. I began to hope that what I learned in my life would be the spark of another's hope, where hope had once been abandoned.

Cancer will beat your hopes into submission, and it will take away so much from your life and those you love. But you can refill, and you can rebuild, and you can regenerate your hope for a life that may be even more profound than your original desires.

Cancer can, and probably will, obliterate your hopes. You can, and hopefully will, rebuild them.

We all find hope where we can, and it is no different with cancer. I found hope in the smallest things. It is amazing how life somehow gives you exactly what you need, exactly when you need it. The following is a simple exchange between Harrison and I via email. I go back to it again and again, and every time it brings me back to those moments when it was that cancer would be nothing more than a brief interruption of all the plans Harrison had made. There is a hope and an innocence in those emails that makes me feel nostalgic. And maybe a little bit angry.

*Hi Sarah-Angel!*

*I hope you are feeling better than you were last night, honey, you were really sick. And I also hope that you slept good, with no nightmares or bad dreams! I have tried calling you a couple of times from my work phone, but you didn't answer, so I guess that means you're sleeping great! It most certainly does not mean that you are ignoring my phone calls...*

*Today totally sucks, because I left my phone at home. I can't believe that I left it. I think it's because I was taking the trash out with me, and I just forgot to pick it up off of the counter, because I already had my wallet and keys in my pocket. It totally sucks, because I am super bored at work today. Normally I check the news on my phone while at work to make the time go by faster, like the CNN app, or USA Today, or Time Mobile. Also I have the Discovery News app, and the G4 app (video gaming news)! But today, regrettably, I don't have my phone, so the day is going by even slower than normal. And the worst news of all is that I can't text my baby angel when she wakes up, and I can't call her on my lunch break!*

*But anyway, I just wanted to let you know that I love you so incredibly much, and no matter what, we are going to get through this. Because I have big plans for us, angel! Marriage, house, kids, vacation trips, all of it! (No cats though, they are most certainly not part of the plan.) You're going to have a great scan on May 2, and they are going to say that you don't need the other treatment. That means that you can come home! That is like 9-10 weeks from today! And 5 weeks from today I'll be there! And I know this summer is going to be tough, honey, and it seems like this battle is never going to end, but it will, honey. We will get you all better by the time school starts, and then you can get back to doing what you love (law school), and living with who you love (ME!!).*

*I love you very much, honey, and I can't wait until you get back home, so that we can get our life back on track! Lots of cuddles, kisses, and other things ;) And dates at Carraba's, Azteca's, and the Thai place!*

*Love You!!*

*Your Harrison*

✦

*Hi Honey!*

*I was so happy to hear from you …*

*I am feeling a little bit better, but my day is going by so slow because you forgot your phone. I didn't realize how much I enjoy our lunch calls until I do not get them anymore :( :( Also, I am sorry for how I was acting last night. I was just really sick and tired. That was a tough chemotherapy, and I pray to God that I never have another one that is like that.*

*Anyway, I talked to professor Fischl and he told me what the three text books are going to be for labor law class and I want to buy them this week. Two of them combined are going to be $80, and then one book is going to $120. I hope it is all right that I need to order these books. We are also meeting in June to go over contracts from the previous semester and discuss everything.*

*I also worked on the Oil & Gas project this morning, which has been a great source of stress, but I feel like we are getting it taken care of. Anyway, I am really looking forward to getting home and getting our life back together. I cannot wait until we can go out on our dinner dates. I think the order for our dates will be 1. Chipotle 2. Carraba's 3. Thai Place and 4. Aztecas. I love all those restaurants and I am excited to try out the new Thai place.*

*More importantly, I am just looking forward to getting my life back on track, and beginning our life together. Without cancer. Also, Mr. Harrison Powers, we are going to get more decorations for the house. I want to get curtains and make our room cuter and not so drab. It is very mannish right now and not cute. If I have to spend a lot of time recovering in there, our place needs a style upgrade. Also, I really enjoy where we live so it looks like we are going to be here for the next three years. I love you, Harrison.*

*Love,*

*Sarah*

# PART THREE

# DYING AND BEYOND

# CHAPTER FIFTEEN

# APPROACHING END OF LIFE CARE

*I will be cremated with my tennis shoes on. That is a nonnegotiable for me. I don't know what is awaiting me on the other side, and just in case the ground is truly hot, I think I will want a pair of shoes.*

✦

I am part of a very small group of stage IV patients who have reached remission or NED state. Whether or how long I will stay is unclear. The treatment I've been through guarantees a new cancer will hit. I just don't know when or how bad it will be. It will always hang over me, but I've found peace with this.

When people find out I have reached NED, they inevitably ask, "Did they catch it early?" I've been asked this question so many times that at this point I have caught myself responding, "Yes, yes," and then have to correct myself and say, "Oh no! It was stage IV." More often than not, when a person first hears stage IV cancer, they see the diagnosis as a death sentence, following up with questions such as, "What is it really like to have stage IV cancer?" and "What does dying feel like?"

In trying to form the most thoughtful and useful response, I always find myself asking in my mind, what does it truly mean to be stage IV?

Looking back, one of the first things that I wish I would've known at the beginning of my diagnosis was that there is a disparity between how early stage and late stage cancer patients are treated. One example occurred when I attended the Look Good Feel Better program, which was a fantastic nonprofit program that helps cancer patients learn beauty techniques in order to help them manage appearance-related side effects. In fact, I enjoyed it so much that I went twice. Both times the program started out with a patient introduction. Similar to how I would assume an Alcoholics Anonymous meeting would go, we would have to stand around the table and one by one go around the room stating our name, diagnosis, and why we were there.

At the first event, which I attended with my sister, we sat next to a mother who had recently been diagnosed with early stage breast cancer and her daughter, who like Alyce, was there for support. My sister and I chatted with them throughout the event, answering as many cancer questions as they asked, and together we laughed as we drew eyebrows onto our faces. A passer-by, unaware of what specifically the event was for, would be justified in thinking it was a women's group luncheon or Junior League meeting. The truth, however, was that the faint echoes of laughter that drifted through the near-empty hospital corridors only served to mask the inescapable truth in each of our eyes, which screamed I don't belong here! Our eyes said could barely contain our desire to jump up and run out of the room sobbing, never looking back.

We were a room full of cancer patients, all putting on our brave and happy faces, trying to feel normal for a night, trying to be grateful to these strangers who seemed to understand how badly we wanted to look like our old healthy selves. But I couldn't help seeing the specter of death in every corner. "Maybe I'll take you," he'd whisper, pointing his sickle at the girl in the black Marc Jacobs dress, "or you," pointing at the young woman with the new engagement ring. I laughed with the women at my table and worked on my makeup tricks, but there was a maniacal edge to it, as if my laughter would keep him from pointing his sickle at me.

A few months later, the mother we chatted with ended up being my younger sister's boss at Microsoft, and she remembered us from the Look Good Feel Better program. I would like to think that some of my sister's good fortune had to do with connecting with the woman at this event. Most people connect over coffee; we just happened to connect over cancer.

By the time I went to my second round of the Look Good Feel Better program, I had learned that it helped to be in the beginning of the pack of patients, as well as early, because this is when most of the best packages were given away. Not all packages were created equal, and I wanted to make sure that I got one of the best! No Mary Kay for me, thanks. Make mine

Chanel! But going first in terms of packages meant going last in terms of awkward icebreakers and introductions.

The majority of the patients who attended these programs were breast cancer patients and had been diagnosed with stage I or stage II breast cancer. Occasionally, there would be other types of cancer—skin, lung, ovarian—it got to be that I could tell who was late stage and who was early by the way they applied their makeup and styled their hair (or lack of it). It was always the eyes.

One thing I learned as a stage IV patient is that I had to be prepared to scare people. I scared my family, my friends, my family, my doctors, and the other patients. Those of us who have given a late stage diagnosis are a pretty exclusive club, and it can be extremely lonely. Nothing can silence a room like a twenty-four-year-old, who looks about thirteen, standing up and saying, "Hello, my name is Sarah, I have stage IVBX refractory Hodgkin lymphoma, and I'm just really excited to learn about the headscarf today!"

Once my diagnosis was out of the bag, it was almost always the same reaction from cancer patients, caregivers, and their friends alike. People would look around the table, begin telling their stories, and then they would qualify their experiences with some variation of the statement, "Now, just let me say that I am not facing anything near what our dear Sarah here is going through, I am sure, but I am Jane Smith…" Every. Single. Time.

Often when someone would say to me, "I'm not saying that it's like anything you went through, that was real cancer," I would get upset. In my mind, cancer was cancer. We were all part of the same horrible group, but apparently there were VIP members and I was the MVP All-Time Hall of Fame Champion.

This is one of the areas in which I would have greatly preferred not to be a VIP who stood out amongst the rest. It made me feel more isolated than I had been before because even among other cancer patients, I was a rare specimen. It became harder and harder to find anyone with whom I could have a real, candid conversation.

In 2013, after moving to Texas for more treatment, still resembling Uncle Fester on his worst day, which was often my best, I had spotted balloons and signs celebrating *Survivors Day!* as Harrison and I drove past the Presbyterian hospital campus here in Dallas, Texas. I was interested in going particularly because I did not know anyone else here in the cancer community, let alone anyone in the community in Texas at all at this point.

I got excited and pleaded with Harrison to take me. He agreed, and we pulled into the parking lot, excited to be celebrating cancer Survivors Day. Worst. Pit stop. Ever.

We made our way through the hospital corridors and entered a room where different items such as orange potted plants, water bottles, T-shirts, and zip drives were displayed. We were early, and I had the whole cornucopia of tchotchkes to choose from. I had enough water bottles, T-shirts were a little too public a statement, and I had collected a drawer full of zip drives from drug companies and doctor's offices over my last three years of treatment. Then I saw the potted plants. I made the argument that because I was young with stage IV cancer, I deserved two potted plants because that's not just one tragedy—it's two. I had just started a flower garden at my new Texas home, and it seemed absolutely necessary that it include a few flowers from Survivors Day. Despite their displeasing aesthetics—unnatural coloration and weed-like foliage—I needed those plants. I mean, they were *survivor* plants. Survivor plants! I needed two, one for each of the identities I wanted to shed: being stage IV and being a young person with cancer. Somehow, it felt as if getting those two plants would change everything. I wouldn't be a tragically young terminal cancer patient. I'd be a *survivor.* A survivor with two ugly plants to prove it.

As other people started funneling into the conference room around me, I was escorted to a specific table toward the front of a room. I looked around, and as the event began, I realized that I may have mistaken cancer Survivors Day, with World War II Survivors Day. I did not see anyone else in the room who was under the age of 70, except for the wait staff. It was extremely uncomfortable, to say the least. Hardly anyone wanted to sit at our table until finally a couple of women sat with us.

As we all chatted, a gentleman, who was wearing a hat and a purple heart-shaped ribbon, approached me and asked, "What are you doing here?

You don't have cancer. You're too young to have cancer. I've never seen you here before, have you been treated here?"

I looked at him and I said, "I do have cancer!"

"No, you don't have cancer. I have cancer, miss. I'm a stage III testicular cancer survivor for thirteen years!"

At that moment, I felt absolutely horrified, and I looked at him indignantly and responded that I was a six-month cancer survivor of stage IV terminal Hodgkin lymphoma.

Finally, in a huff, he turned and walked away. As we were waiting for the program to begin, I suddenly realized all these people had been treated at the Presbyterian hospital except for me. I was the outlier because, thank my good graces, I was treated at Stanford. Harrison and I nervously wondered if this was a Presbyterian-patients-only event. We were quickly reassured that it wasn't by the only other stage IV cancer survivor in the room. She'd had a brain tumor that had left her disabled in terms of her vision as well as her hearing. Even though she was only in her 50s, she could no longer drive or walk by herself because her vision and equilibrium were no longer adequate for her to navigate on her own. She'd chosen to sit with me.

This woman, when we went around the table and told our stories, was heartbroken and felt sorry for me. The woman with the malignant brain tumor, who couldn't even stand up without wobbling over, felt sorry for me.

I walked away from the event with my two plants and a waffle maker I won in the closing raffle. It ended up being a pretty good electronic flat-iron waffle maker. I can just plug it into the wall and throw some batter onto it, and have waffles in about five seconds. I imagine I'll use this once I am bedridden and can't actually use the telephone to order my food directly for myself. Should this day ever come, my friend Courtney Sermone will unplug me or Kevorkian me, whichever one comes easiest. Then she can eat my waffles.

✦

After I was admitted to Stanford, just prior to my stem cell transplant, I had a roommate whose idea of a good time was comparing the personal cancer atrocities we had suffered. It was a strange competition where the winner, I am assuming, as set out by my roommate's terms of the game, would be the one who had the deadlier diagnosis. It reminded me of watching fraternity brothers, mediocre co-workers, and even rival executives engage in one-upping each other in normal aspects of life. I was surprised and found it a bit morbid and disturbing that this was also a pastime in the cancer world.

She won.

By a landslide.

I requested to be transferred to a private room.

✦

One of the first things that I noticed that made me different as a stage IV cancer patient was that I couldn't have cared less about losing my hair. It was a shock and seemed like a waste of all the time I'd spent growing my hair out and maintaining its health for so many years. But it didn't tweak my vanity. As doctor after nurse after social worker expressed sympathy and even empathy for the fact that I was going to (and eventually did) lose my hair, I just kept thinking, "Is this really what you think the problem is?" I had more medical care professionals address how I felt about the loss of my hair than ever addressed how I felt about the very likely loss of my life.

I know hair loss is a very important issue especially for women who tie up their femininity and self-identity with their hair. I have read many cancer books, and this issue about hair loss is always addressed, but it is one that I just never quite found myself being able to empathize with all that much. I suppose at some point it can be extremely hard for a woman to lose her hair because of chemotherapy and radiation. I suppose it can be a visual reminder of the illness that is hard on a lot of patients. But that was absolutely the last thing I was concerned about when I was losing my life. Once I realized my life was on the line, my hair became unimportant. Cancer took so much more away from me than my hair. I wasn't going to make that another internal traumatizing struggle, so I just shaved my hair off and yelled good riddance.

✦

While not everyone with terminal cancer worries about how they look, I have found that we all worry about how we will die. It's a subject that at once terrifies people and fills them with curiosity. People like me, whose appearance screamed cancer, have their boundaries stripped away. Some of it is necessity (doctors and nurses and techs must do what is best for a patient's health, not what is best for avoiding embarrassment). But a lot of it is just strangers wanting to guard themselves against cancer by arming themselves with all the ways they are unlike the patient.

Every terminal patient has people actively planning for their passing. Not just medical professionals either. I had a number of these types of individuals. They made their role clear because they never talked about me, my life, or my cancer treatment, in the present tense. They did not engage in the tyranny of cheerfulness, nor did they advocate for my fight against the scourge of cancer. It was refreshing because I didn't have to put on the "smile or die" attitude. I didn't have to fake it to make other people comfortable with my disease. It got so exhausting having to do that everyday with my family that when I met someone that I could be real and honest with, it was like I could breathe again.

I am not an advocate of sticking one's head in the sand when it comes to the subject of death. But people with cancer still have boundaries. I never knew quite how to react to people who started to ask me about my religious preferences upon death completely out of the blue. They'd ask about my thoughts on the afterlife and where I believed I'd be going, whether I would like to be cremated or buried, and if I was afraid of what would happen when I died.

Despite all the good things social networking has brought to cancer patients, it has done nothing to encourage boundaries. When my cancer became public knowledge (my baldness was the giveaway) I received a ton of Facebook messages. Most of them were encouraging, many were panicked, and a few were incredibly invasive. One message came from a girl I had gone to school with many years ago and could hardly remember. Along with the questions about my cancer and my beliefs, which I had not considered at the time, was her request for forgiveness for a number of things that I could not even recall. Like all good popes and Catholics do, I forgave her for all the supposed ills that she thought she had brought against me. But I couldn't help to wonder why she hadn't apologized long before.

A lot of people have a morbid fascination with death. And terminal cancer patients draw them like bees to flowers. It can be unnerving. These people start to ask questions about the patient's death in the most random of places. They ask for the most intimate details of the patient's life and beliefs. Not only that, they are the most random of people. I'm talking about the grocery clerk at the local Knob Hill, the cashier at the movie theater, and even the nurse at the local blood bank. For these people, a bald head and pale skin is an invitation.

When I was first diagnosed with terminal cancer in 2012, I learned that time on earth was brief. Most of us have been asked at one time or another what we would do if we were given six months to live. It's usually just a harmless game, a frame by which we can explore what is truly important in our lives. Most people's answers include some variation of an island, margaritas, and skydiving. However, the reality is, when we are put in that situation for real, we have one choice to make and it has nothing to do with which island to visit first. It is whether or not to begin cancer treatment and risk spending the last months of life receiving chemotherapy, radiation, surgeries, experimental treatments, and rolling the dice in clinical trials. Or not. It's an issue of quality versus quantity.

Some people choose not to get cancer treatment and would rather spend their last without the devastating effects that these treatments cause. We have the choice of suffering through treatment in hopes of extending our lives, or forego treatment and feel like ourselves as long as we can. A terminal cancer diagnosis does not sugarcoat the consequences of our decisions. When patients choose to not go through treatment, they know they are living out what ultimately are the last days of their lives. With cancer, inaction *is* action.

✦

One of the biggest issues a terminal diagnosis brings is when to start entering the end-of-life care phase. It is a deeply personal, often frightening, and complex issue that will color the patient's future decisions. Some patients take the mortality issue and choose to live life in the moment, leaving future concerns and plans on the side and approaching life day by day. Others will actively plan for the future. Examples of this are setting up wills, funeral arrangements, and getting financial affairs in order. It is common for patients facing a terminal illness to replace trying to accomplish personal goals with attending milestone events such as graduations, weddings, or the birth of a grandchild. It becomes more important to experience and be present for these momentous occasions, than reaching a personal goal.

For terminal patients, counseling is often recommended, and religious patients may request religious figures of their choosing to come and assist them with end of their life. In my experience, the patients who hold some sort of religious belief or a belief in an afterlife face a terminal diagnosis with less anxiety and fear.

However, not all end-of-life issues are philosophical. There are plenty of concrete details that need to be addressed. .

Which funeral home or mortuary do you want your body to be taken to after you pass away?

Most people don't think about this. It will likely be one that was chosen by relatives who have gone before you and will likely have been a funeral home that your loved ones have worked with and know. Now, that's not necessarily a bad choice and could be, in fact, a very good choice if you do have a family history with a particular funeral home. However, I do caution the discerning patient to visit the funeral home or mortuary for oneself. Having visited several funeral homes and mortuaries through my time, I know they can differ greatly.

Do you want to be embalmed? Buried? Cremated?

I myself will not be embalmed despite my fiancé's attempts to possibly stuff me and nail me to a wall like a lion here in Texas. I will be cremated. I will be cremated with my tennis shoes on. That is a nonnegotiable for me. I don't know what is awaiting me on the other side, and just in case the ground is truly hot, I think I will want a pair of shoes.

Who would you like to have notified of your death?

If you happen to be someone who either is extremely famous or per-haps someone who has spent the majority of life in elected isolation, then a list like this may be something useful. For those of us without any particular notoriety, people are going to figure out on their own that we've died. For most of us, we don't need to have a mass mailing list go out to notify our hordes of fans, nor do we need to hire a private investigator to find our one friend from second grade who we wish to notify of our passing.

Who's going to write the eulogy? Can I suggest an answer? You should write your own. I have written my own eulogy to avoid some of the language that really irks me. No one is going to say I lost my *battle* with the scourge of cancer.

You need to think about where you are going to be buried or, if you're going to be cremated, where you would like your ashes to be scattered? Would you like them to be in an urn? Myself, I will be cremated and scattered among the meadow in which my grandmother has herself been scattered. Sometimes people like to keep a little reminder of their past loved ones by keeping a portion of ashes in an urn, or in my grandmother's case, a Costco cookie jar.

If you're planning on getting a burial plot, you want to consider whether or not you want headstone or grave marker. Think carefully about what you want to have inscribed on your headstone or grave marker. This is literally the last statement you will leave the world. I suggest you think about this thoroughly, as I am relatively certain you would not want it to say, "Dan was here."

The two most common types of end-of-life festivities are a funeral service and a funeral program, the latter being more formal. You're going to want to choose which one you would prefer. I myself will be having a funeral service. If you have any particular needs for the ceremonies, such as you are member of the military or you have particular religious preferences, you're going to want to discuss those in advance.

Who will deliver your eulogy? Choose carefully here. This person will be recapping your life's work, importance, and impact on the world for what may be the last time. Do you really want people to recount that time in the sixth grade when you and your friend Joe went and stole rock candy bars from the 7-Eleven and got drunk on nonalcoholic beer?

Now, for myself because, I will likely be dying relatively young, I will want Harrison to read a section of my eulogy, which I will have prewritten, and next have my mother read a prewritten section of my eulogy, and last will have a wildcard selection.

✦

Being young, and prior to my diagnosis, a relatively healthy and vivacious individual, I didn't have any person in my life—despite the great wealth of love and support I had—with whom I was able to have a serious and realistic discussion with regarding my end-of-life care and final wishes. In the end, these were all factors that I sorted out alone after visiting hours were over, when my room grew silent and dark. I ended up giving my end-of-life instructions to a nurse.

It wasn't for a lack of trying. There were multiple times when I tried, at times desperately, to raise these issues with my mother or with Harrison, but the idea or even the discussion of my death was literally unspeakable. This only worsened as my condition became increasingly dire.

It was in the very real sense, very similar to the story of Voldemort and *Harry Potter.* Death was my "he who shall not be named." The conversation about death and dying quickly became a toxic issue that if discussed out loud, many people literally believed, just may induce the very thing we were trying to prevent: my death.

The only time I've actually seen people who believe that speaking certain words out-loud would induce a particular dramatic or tragic outcome would be on the paranormal reality shows on my favorite channel, Lifetime. What I have learned from my highly technical and respected paranormal education is that in dealing with the paranormal (or really anything not in a science book) is the idea that when a person discusses anything negative or painful, those negative energies and entities will attach to that person and manifest, feeding off the negative attention. Yet how many of you reading here would agree that this is something you absolutely believe to be true? I'm guessing not many. However, it is overwhelmingly common, and almost certain and predictable, that even the most rational people will take this type of belief structure and approach, and apply it to discussions on death and dying. Hence, Voldemort.

When I was a very young child, around the age of three or four, I believed that at night when I was scared of the dark, if I could not see the monsters when I closed my eyes, that they could not see me. This made complete sense to my three-year-old mind, but as I grew up I learned differently.

You can imagine what it was like when I was approaching the point where I needed to discuss the practical aspects of my death, and every person covered their eyes, turned away, and shunned the monster. But I felt as if by turning away and covering their eyes, they were turning away from me as their loved one, unable to continue with me through this very difficult process.

I think of a quote from Shakespeare's *Henry V,* written in 1598, quite frequently, "Once more unto the breach, dear friends, once more" and then I think about how in reality, the majority of people react in these types of death and dying situations more like, "Once more unto the breach, dear friends, once more; until shit gets real, and then you're on your own." You're left to march off that cliff by yourself.

Remember, when we do pass, we can't take anyone with us. So get comfortable and find some peace and stability. Seek solace within your own soul and in your own person, because that is the one who is going to be holding your hand when you cross the great divide.

# CHAPTER SIXTEEN

# ON DEATH AND DYING

*We don't know our breaking point until we break.*

✦

It is my dream that I live the rest of my days with intention and purpose, in the hope that as I die with eyes wide open the time I spend until I reach that point is time my loved ones will get what they need in terms of preparation and opportunity to say goodbye. I hope they will be in a place where they are closer to coming to peace with my death and the hand I was dealt knowing that not a moment was wasted. I want to die well, and it is my highest hope for my loved ones that they have some semblance of closure and that they go on to live full and flourishing lives.

"In the darkness... Lord, my God, who am I that you should forsake me? The child of your love – and now become as the most hated one. The one – you have thrown away as unwanted – as unloved. I call, I cleaned, I want, and there is no one to answer... Where I tried to raise my thoughts to heaven, there is such convicting emptiness that those very thoughts return like sharp knives and hurt my very soul. Love – the word – it brings nothing. I am told God lives in me – and yet the reality of darkness and coldness and emptiness is so great that nothing touches my soul." – Mother Theresa, 1957

✦

I have seen cancer rip through families with a speed and stealth that is unimaginable. I've seen many caregivers walk away and abandon their loved ones. In the end, many of us find that to truly love brings a great burden. With great love comes great suffering and pain. It often requires us to see past momentary situations or feelings that can be fleeting, in adherence to a belief in a love greater than the case at hand, even if that love is not present for us to grab onto or to rest our heads upon, or for us to call on in the hour of our greatest need. To love greatly is to sacrifice oneself for another. I have seen cancer cripple love. I have seen cancer shine the light of truth upon what was once thought a great love, but which upon its meeting with cancer, proved to be rather dim and conditional. I have seen cancer bring men and women to the brink of their capacity to truly love, only to find that their ability to love was in itself not strong enough, not great enough, and not, in itself, enough to withstand the of challenges of such an all-encompassing illness.

Cancer can cripple love. Cancer *does* cripple love. Cancer has crippled my life's great love. While cancer did not abolish this love, it was crippled and came just a breath away from a complete loss. I held on to this love of mine, grasping for any hope that it might still retain just a glimmer of what it once was before cancer. We are still building.

But in the darkness and chaos of an unreconciled mind circling and twisting the broken fragments of a life lost, in the labyrinth of false truths weaved together with misguided reason and the logic of an untouched mind, dwelled the grace of God.

In the moments of silence in this chaotic mind weary from the relentless stream of thought and racing rationalizations spiraling as if on fire, did in those rare moments of silence and peace when I could think no more, with nothing more than a whisper; the soul did speak.

It was then that I overcame death, and I was transformed.

✦

When I received my cancer diagnosis and knew just how far and aggressively my cancer had spread, I immediately began the reconciling of my soul. It was one of the darkest moments of my life. I struggled considerably not only with my physical death but with what I had done in my life and what I had not. The point that broke me, the greatest pain I have ever endured, was having to accept that in death, the person I was then was the highest form of self that I would have achieved in this life.

I always wanted to be a person of high integrity and character, a person who made wise decisions and chose to act because it was the right thing to do, always. At that point in my life, it was so easy for me to continue living my life with a particular set of personality traits that had made me very successful. But was that really me?

I feared I would die without ever having been true to who I really was. Would I walk away from what came so easily, and have the courage to live my life accordingly? I was the source of a lot of pain for others, and there were times when I inspired such great feelings of ill will, I scared myself. When I say that I had to reconcile with my soul, it is to say that I had to face the hard truth that in life I had lived my life as a coward, a masked person too afraid or too vapid to act in accordance with my real self.

By the middle of July 2012, I was beginning to slide into what was the direst condition. August was full of extreme pain as well as horrible, traumatic experiences with the various medications and chemotherapies, which induced severe side effects. But the physical side of cancer was not the hardest thing I dealt with during those dark days.

✦

We don't know our own breaking point until we break. This time in my life tested me fully. My character, my faith, and my integrity would eventually call upon me to forgive and even understand, which I still struggle with immensely.

My life with Harrison at the time of my cancer diagnosis and treatment, challenged us until our foundation crumbled. This is how cancer finally broke me, and every day I continue to pray to God for the strength to rise stronger in these broken places.

When I was first diagnosed. Harrison and I were living in Connecticut, and I was studying law at the University of Connecticut. Harrison, by that December, was working for a large financial firm headquartered on the east coast. The prior six months leading up to my diagnosis, Harrison was looking for the perfect job, and I supported us as I worked sixty-hour work weeks with the firm Turner & Townsend. I was working out of our home in Connecticut and going to the New York office when necessary—all while also attending law school full-time. I will note that I have an unusually high capacity for what most people consider large amounts of work, and I managed to do both quite well. This schedule was my choice, because what I wanted most was for Harrison to be able to find a career with one firm with which he could build a long and successful career.

He found this position, this career we had been holding out for, in November 2011. It was such a short time from when he started and got settled to when cancer would thrash and rip our lives apart at the very seams. In the beginning, I was relentless in holding onto the non-negotiable fact that I would be returning to our home in Connecticut immediately following any treatment. I continued to work full-time with Turner & Townsend remotely from chemotherapy infusion clinics, hospitals, and from my home in Nevada in bed curled up after a round of chemotherapy.

Harrison made the decision to remain on the east coast. To keep things together at our home in Connecticut, and I suppose that my decision to continue working without fail or informing any of my colleagues that I had been diagnosed with cancer, made it not only financially possible to maintain our home but it was also a tangible link to the life I loved so dearly.

I am often asked if Harrison went through those couple of years by my side and the general truth is that yes, he did. However, he was not, for the majority, physically present. Yes, we had Skype and FaceTime to communicate, but as for having him near to hold my hand when I was afraid or in pain, he was not. It was not until it became apparent just how ill I was and that I would die in the upcoming months or even weeks that Harrison stayed with me. For the first seven months of my cancer treatment, Harrison remained in Connecticut. We had become accustomed to a particular income and lifestyle, and I think in part because of that it was difficult for him to finally make the decision to leave Connecticut.

At the point in May 2012 when my cancer was found to be refractory to the front-line chemotherapy regimen ABVD, I relapsed and was again dying very quickly. When Harrison got the news, he resigned from his dream position and packed up our home in Connecticut and placed our things in storage in Dallas, Texas, where his family lived. He came out to a vacation home my parents' had rented in Half Moon Bay, California, where I was staying to be close to Stanford. He was with me as my primary caregiver for five months, which was the absolute limit of his ability to cope.

As I became increasingly ill following my bone marrow transplant on September 3, 2012, my mother and Harrison seemed to constantly bicker regarding my medical care, even over my medications and the dosages. My mom believed that Harrison coddled me and needed to be firmer and show tough love when I refused to get up, walk around, or even do simple leg presses from my hospital bed. They were both living at the vacation house and all the time together was weighing on their relationship. By the time I was well enough to join them at the home, things were pretty thoroughly off the rails between them.

My mother hated the way the medications changed my typically very assertive and outgoing personality, and she fought for a decrease in my medication. She never backed down, be it with the nurses, my doctors, or Harrison and the arguments soon turned into something that happened on a daily basis.

At one point I was lightly dozing, not comatose, when my mother tried to assert power of attorney over me, claiming that I was incapable of making my own decisions because my mental capacities were diminished significantly by the drugs. The psychiatrist who had prescribed many of the medications was no match for my mother. He finally agreed.

Well, I am my mother's daughter, and I'll never forget how quickly my ass popped out of that hospital bed and declared aggressively, "The only person who may legally make decisions over my healthcare is me. If any physician on this team does so without my explicit written consent, unless I am actually incapacitated, I will sue every person on this medical team for failure to act in accordance with the law if they grant power of attorney over my person every time I take a goddamn nap."

Then, I lay back down, hit the morphine pump, and went back to sleep. I was told later that my psychiatrist was extremely proud in that moment. Needless to say, my mother did not get power of attorney over my person that day.

Following the transplant, because of my relentless, stubborn refusal to walk, I developed a severe lung infection. Fluid was building up in my lungs faster than it was draining and quickly the bacterial infection spread throughout my chest. This prolonged my stay in the hospital for more than a month. I could no longer walk or even hold myself up, let alone hold a book up to read, so I got all my books in audio files and kept my mind from wandering into increasing temptation of just letting myself finally pass. I was like a drunk driver falling asleep at the wheel, slapping myself to keep awake just long enough to get home safely, without collateral damage and alive.

I was lucky that my parents had rented the vacation home. While my doctors would not have been comfortable with my going all the way home to Nevada between treatments, they allowed me to stay in California. Harrison was there. It was about mid-October, and all of the Halloween decorations and pumpkins were coming out. I remember the pumpkin patches so vividly. It is a warm memory, but a fleeting one. I immediately began high dose targeted radiation therapy that would last months, five days a week, no break in treatment, not even for Christmas.

I was only there for a few months but that time is vivid in my memory. I loved the beach there because it was always cool and foggy. The colors seemed to be so strong and the drive those days to and from the hospital were beautiful along those windy roads. I think that is why my mother chose that house for that time. It was a beautiful place for me to be where all the things I love about nature were spread before me.

But during this time, my mother and Harrison's relationship was becoming increasingly strained. Harrison spent little if any time with me, unlike he had at the beginning of our time at Half Moon Bay, watching movies and giggling about who wore it better, me or Uncle Fester. (Fester always won.) He became extremely irritated and quickly put on edge. He started to spend all of his time in the cave-like gaming room. I tried my best, begging and begging for him to tell me what was wrong, terrified it was something I'd done. He never loved me any less, but his capacity for love was met. He gave everything that he could, and that was those five months. Nothing more, nothing less.

On the morning of November 19, like most mornings, I was lying in my bed unable to do much except turnover and take my medications. At this point, even taking a shower was an Olympic race, so even that was rare. Nevertheless, every morning I felt Harrison's body next to mine when I awoke, and it gave me a deep peace and calm.

One morning I awoke early. It was about five o'clock, and I instinctively sought out Harrison's body next to mine. There was nothing. While I slept, Harrison had packed his things, kissed me very lightly on the forehead, and left. He never even hesitated or turned around for even just a single moment; he did not stop until he reached Dallas, Texas, his hometown where he was going to start again.

When I woke up, and found Harrison was gone, I completely abandoned for the first time in my life. There was no hope or love, and even God and my faith were absent. It was a pain like I had never felt before. It was the pain of having my entire being ripped from my bones and left raw with great loss and darkness. There was nothing but a complete void.

It was not until I seriously began studying theology and was taken in by the beautiful loving souls at the Highland Park United Methodist Church in Dallas, Texas, several years later that I would come across the only writings that could express this devastating period of my life through the letters of Mother Teresa. I cried the first time during ministry when I heard her words read out loud. It was terrible to learn of the anguish that Mother Teresa experienced for so long during her lifetime, but I also broke down crying because this was the void that consumed my life. For Mother Teresa, God's love and presence were entirely absent. For about twenty years, she battled with the feeling of God's absence in her life. This was revealed in her letters after her death and her discussions on her experiences with the spiritual phenomenon of the dark night of the soul. It was darkness. It is darkness. It is just complete darkness.

My father explained to me that Harrison had left because he didn't expect me to live. He didn't think I would be meeting up with him in Dallas in the future to start a life there, and he was young and just wanted to go home. Harrison never defended himself against that statement nor did he ever have any guilt or remorse about leaving me during the most crucial time when I was at my most vulnerable.

✦

When Harrison wasn't present while I was in the hospital for treatment I was more understanding because I was often heavily medicated. I acknowledged that it was not necessary for him to be there, because there would be nothing much for him to do. However, it was impossible for me to justify him leaving me alone at the cancer center when I was facing certain death. Then, in what felt like cruel irony, I survived. I was forced to learn to live again in the most primal and basic ways.

I had to learn how to walk again. I had to learn how to control my bowel muscles again. Like a baby, I wore diapers for months. I was so ill that I had to wear a large gas-mask-like breathing filter twenty-four hours a day to block out impurities. Thank God that it came in pink. There I was at 25, wearing diapers, unable to walk, wearing a pink gas mask, bald, and with no eyebrows or eyelashes. At this point, I was so absurd looking that just one glance at me would put any cancer commercial to shame.

When I was dying in the hospital, Harrison had started to become very distant, and I could tell that he was getting sick and tired of me being sick and tired. This, however, was not enough for me to be able to come to a place where I can say I forgave his actions when he left me. This brutal moment right before I was forced to get up and learn to survive again, with this horrible decrepit and fractured body, I needed him.

When I started walking again, it was one of the most painful things I'd ever experienced because my muscles had atrophied to the point where they barely existed. My muscles were hardly functioning, and they reacted when I would simply walk up and down stairs. The tears in the muscle movement caused lactic acid to seep in to begin to rebuild the muscle. This caused excruciating pain.

Harrison took me to the beach once at Half Moon Bay. He drove me, of course. It was a cloudy day and the fog was heavy, but I managed to get out of the car and stand on my own and walk over to the sand. I can still remember for the first time I really cried because I never ever thought I would ever feel a breeze again or see the ocean (my most favorite place in the whole world), let alone feel the sand on my skin. I wanted to stay there forever despite how cold it was (and it was freezing). Half Moon Bay at that time of year was foggy and dreary but that was exactly my perfect idea of what a beach is. No one was there but us. We didn't talk much at all. If we did, I don't remember what was said. I remember I wanted to stay so badly, but it was getting colder and the breeze was really picking up, and Harrison had to get me back to the house because I wasn't supposed to be out in the elements, but I had my pink gas mask on so I could be there for a short while. There was a house on the edge of the shore on a cliff, and I remember thinking, *one day I am going to live there.* Who knows maybe I still will.

✦

Family members and friends stopped visiting. I stopped interacting with anyone on a day-to-day basis because just the sight of me caused them so much pain. The only thing I could do was to try and give back to my family and the people I loved a sense of normalcy in their lives, and this meant doing my best to avoid having them look at me in this condition.

I stopped getting out of bed, and I would listen to my mother whistling like she had before our lives were affected by cancer. She told me once that at that time she would be outside riding her horses and would catch herself in a moment of happiness, almost forgetting it all, even just for one moment. I loved the thought of this. I wanted her to sing and whistle and ride her horses and be the beautiful, vibrant light she always radiated. I knew that these moments for her were brief and fleeting, and it took just one glance back at the house for her to remember her cancer-ridden daughter tucked away. She told me she always felt guilty if she felt any moments of joy, and this broke my heart because she was my entire happiness and the light of my life. The worst thing about dying a slow, long death from cancer is watching the people you love so dearly watch you die.

The family who was once very close wouldn't even come into the house if they knew I was awake because they said it was too painful for them to see me. It was when it became too painful for the people that I loved, who had been such an important part of my life to just look at me that I wished that I would've died one hundred times to spare them the anguish that was so clear in their pained faces.

I know that I am not going to be able to go through what I went through a second time, and when the time comes for me to cross over the great divide, I want to go alone. I want to go knowing my family will carry on with their lives and that my passing will not be crippling. Especially for my mother. I want the world for her; I only want to see her happy and hear her whistling from the barn up to the birds. I will do everything I can to give her every moment like this, up to my last breath. She will never have to watch her daughter dying again because that is too much pain for any mother to have to bear.

*(September 2012)*

*Hey, Mom!*

*You should see this place!*

*Now, I want to quickly clear up some serious misconceptions for you so that when you arrive here in Heaven, you don't think you made a wrong turn and that the light you walked into was from a pair of headlights on a speeding car. Trust me, it happens all the time, making it impossible to keep any reasonable schedule for business hours! Do not worry, you know me, I was on it the minute I got here! This should be taken care of by the time you and dad get here.*

*First, when you walk into the light, it is nothing like how my favorite Lifetime Paranormal episodes made it out to be. There is no dark figure to guide you through or some strange mass floating toward you. If you think this through, hiring a guide for every single person who comes in is a horrible use of funds. Really, it is a tunnel of light now, isn't it? Where else are you going to go?! It is not a fork in the road, and it is too late to turn around and ask for directions because well, that ship has sailed.*

*Second, remember that a tunnel of light is not a wormhole. This is not Star Gate, so do not be disappointed when you do not fly through the galaxies of space, and wake up inside of a Pyramid in Egypt.*

*Third, you are going to be nervous when you get here. It is almost like going to court because you did not pay your parking tickets. It's Judgment Day!! However, don't worry, everyone, including you will be scared to death and looking for any upside to Hell that you can think of because you are thinking that there is absolutely no way you're getting in after you "borrowed" that nickel from your mom's purse when you were five. You know who you are.*

*Finally, let me save you from this rookie mistake and further explain a couple of important details. There is no resemblance of anything "pearly" or even a gate, for that matter. This is not My Little Pony meets the Federal Reserve, and to put it bluntly, if you are adamantly looking for the "pearly gates of heaven," you will wander forever. Fun fact: that is precisely how Paranormal Activity began! No one is a damned soul seeking redemption for their sins; they are just lost with bad directions.*

*Furthermore, the apostle Paul is not sitting in judgment as you all stand in line like a DMV clerk as he checks you off his naughty or nice list. He is not Santa Claus. That would be irrational; we all know Santa Clause does not exist. However, this did give us a good idea for April Fool's Day next year. We are all just waiting for the third member of the holy trinity to figure out his schedule. He is picked up some bad habits from his time on earth, which I blame on his twelve closest buddies—disciples of the Lord, I think not!*

*Also, this will interest you. You know the guy who owns this place is kind of a big deal. It was a long time ago—before your time—but in His prime, He was the one who created the universe, and rumor has it that He did it in seven days. Well, He says that supposedly, He finished the project in an impressive six, on time and within budget. Then He did not have anything left to do on the seventh day, so He took the day off.*

*He preaches being humble about His accomplishments, so, He does not bother to correct anyone, but we all know He was sleeping on the seventh day. Very humble, my Lord. . A couple of us up here got suspicious about this, and me and apostle John snuck into double-check His credentials to make sure that we hadn't been duped into taking the exit for damnation instead of exaltation. I also secretly double-checked to make sure I didn't die on April 1st, and that there was no April Fool's prank, because I was the April Fool's prank!*

*I love it here, Mom. Do you remember when you sent me to summer camp year after year, and I was always the one child that never ever wanted it to end? It is a little like that. We even get field trips, to visit loved ones, and even have super powers that let us see everything! It is fantastic!*

*I know that right now this letter feels like a knife in your heart, but I promise that there will come a day when the pain will be less, and you will pick this letter up again, but this time it won't be drenched with your tears, and it won't break your heart. I promise you one day you will read this with a smile, and you may even laugh. There is so much of my personality and spirit in these words that you never have to be afraid of forgetting as the years start to pass, and memories fade.*

*Well, mom, this is it. We have finally come full circle now. I know that right now you do not think you will survive this and are scared to death to let me go. Right now, you are with the family and about to spread my ashes in the meadow with Grandma's. Before you do, I want you to step away for a minute so that I can say goodbye the best way I can.*

*At this moment, I am right beside you. Although I will no longer be physically present, I am with you every moment from the second you wake up in the morning to when you fall asleep at night. I am in the light of the sun whose warmth comforts you, even on your darkest days. I am atop the snow-capped mountains watching over you always, knowing that I am home. You will hear my voice in the cool crisp breeze that runs through the evergreens, the rhythm of the glistening bustling creek, and in the sweet song of the birds. My beauty and soul are in everything that surrounds you and my spirit plays among the vibrant wildflowers dancing across this meadow. Know that I am beside you now and that you will never be without me. Simply look to the light of the sun and feel the warmth it brings or gaze up at the brightest star in the sky, and I promise you will see me there. Always.*

*What a beautiful life! The adventures we had, full of laughter and more "once in a lifetime moments" than any person could ever wish. The time we had could fill a thousand lifetimes. Never forget that.*

*I love you, mom.*

# CHAPTER SEVENTEEN

# ON SURVIVORSHIP

*I was extremely blessed that I made the two-year milestone NED without recurrence. It felt as if some warmongering madman had finally taken his hand off the nuclear launch button.*

✦

When I learned I would survive cancer, my family celebrated, and I cried. Eventually, people stopped tiptoeing around me or hugging me for just a little bit too long at dinner parties. Friends stopped saying "goodbye" and started saying "see you later" once again. Everyone it seemed was able to pick up right where they left off with their lives without a second thought. Everyone but me.

The last thing I wanted was to dwell on that state and keep others there with me. Nothing was as it had been before cancer. I was not the same person as I was, and if I was to come successfully out of my experience stronger in the places I had been broken, I had to learn to live beyond cancer.

Inevitably, cancer patients and survivors will have some degree of fear regarding the recurrence of their cancer. In the more severe cases, patients with high anxiety regarding recurrence can be slower to return to a productive lifestyle out of nervousness their cancer could return. It can cause mental paralysis and prevent the patient from making plans and "moving on" with their life. While we often cannot eliminate the fear of recurrence, we can learn how to cope with the fear in a way that does not prevent us from having an active, productive lifestyle.

Don't try to manage your fears alone. You can try joining a support group for other cancer survivors where you can talk about your concerns. But you can also talk to a close friend or relative about how you are feeling. If you're too embarrassed to discuss your anxieties out loud, try writing about them in a journal to help you express yourself.

Maintain a healthy post-cancer lifestyle. Try to eat healthy meals and exercise, and also be careful to adhere to your doctor's follow-up care regimen. Most cancers have studied rates of recurrence, and your doctor can help keep you educated about the rates and the best ways to avoid recurrence.

Try to find ways to reduce your anxiety and stress levels. Find time to relax and do things you enjoy. Find time for humorous activities and things that make you laugh. Don't overschedule yourself and say yes to every activities but do say yes to going out with friends. Get help with financial burdens such as medical debt that may cause excess anxiety (apply for grants, apply for assistance through the government, apply for hospital financial aid for qualifying patients, major cancer organizations such as the American Cancer Society, advocacy organizations such as Stupid Cancer, raise funds using social media on GoFundMe). Find a cancer support group or help hotline to help you talk about how you're feeling.

On September 3, 2014, I reached my two-year bone marrow post-transplant milestone. Reaching the two-year milestone was something I believed I would never live to see. But I didn't trust I was NED. I'd spent the last two years preparing for death and living from treatment to treatment. Regardless of how I felt or what the doctors said, I needed a clean PET scan before I would relax at all. I awaited the schedule date on pins and needles.

Certain that this would be the PET scan that would inevitably show that cancer had returned to plunge me back into the grips of the bone marrow transplant unit, I was as concerned and anxious as ever. I was terrified that I would be tucked away in that same corner hospital room with the butterflies and pink bubblegum wallpaper until my untimely death. However, this time it was a bit different. I also had anxiety about what I would do if I did not have a recurrence. I found that I was just as terrified that I would live to an old age as I was that I would re-enter treatment.

I was extremely blessed that I made the two-year milestone without recurrence. It felt as if some warmongering madman had finally taken his hand off the nuclear launch button. In fact, I never knew how dire and uncertain my medical teams were until after I made the milestone; you could hear the collective sigh of relief from all the doctors from California to Texas.

I wish I could tell you that I have found my fear of recurrence has subsided over the past two years since I was declared NED, but that has not been my experience. There's not a day that goes by that I do not think about cancer recurrence. I live knowing that the life I have built could be taken away with just one scan. I live my life in six-month increments as I am re-adjusting and coming to terms with my experience.

Living from PET scan to PET scan, it took quite a while before I would allow myself to entertain the idea of seriously planning for a family of my own. Finally discussing retirement plans with Harrison. Allowing myself to argue about where our love bench would go in the front yard—which we sat on every evening, waving at the neighbors as they arrived home from work.

Harrison proposed on December 23, 2013, in South Africa. But planning for an event almost a year away feels foreign and unattainable. While my rational mind tells me that I will live to see my wedding day, I can't say to you in truth that I believe that I will.

Most of my colleagues are planning what's next on the ladder to the top and how many rungs to climb and hoops they will need to run through to get there. Many people find me a bit unnerving or out of place in this race to nowhere. They think I have some special secret as if I have unlocked the key to success and am withholding it to gain the upper hand. The honest truth is that I have just stopped running, planning, and working myself into an early grave because the chances of relapse were high and this forced me to live in the present moment.

Cancer has caused me to re-evaluate what I consider a good life. I have learned for myself, a good life is one lived with intention, acute awareness, and directed energy. It is most fulfilling for me when I spend the time I have been given in a channeled, focused way. I have priorities but by priorities, I do not mean ten urgent things all vying for my attention. I keep my priorities narrow—one, maybe two. Three at most. Furthermore, one of them is me!

For the first time in my life, I've made myself a priority. I make sure to get enough sleep, to take long walks, and get out into nature. I've tried to eat a more balanced diet and forgive myself for the extra five pounds. I've allowed myself to put my well being before the rat race, money, and social status. These are no longer priorities in my life, but I had to give myself the permission to let them fall aside and put myself first. In doing this, I've had to become comfortable with the uncertainty that comes with surviving cancer, and I'm finally taking it in stride. I am still learning and have a long way to go on the second phase of my journey, but so far I like where I am headed.

I am still learning how to live beyond treatment on a fundamental level. I am taking it day by day. I'm learning how my body now functions—as an entirely different structure. I have different limitations and physical requirements that I didn't have before I was diagnosed. I am learning how to give myself time. I am also rediscovering new and amazing things about myself every day. Yes, it is challenging. Yes, it is difficult and frustrating many days. But, yes, it is exhilarating at the same time because I am constantly discovering new things about my perspectives, passions, and purposes each day.

In a nutshell, this is the tough stuff. You don't have to hate cancer; you don't have to curse it each time someone with a pink ribbon comes around the corner. It has been my experience that those who do best are the ones who don't dwell on it and do not give it any more time than it has already taken away from them. That includes the time one spends thinking about it while stopped at a traffic light.

Allow yourself to accept what is and what is not, and give yourself permission to let go of pieces of who you once were but no longer are. Get to know yourself as you are now, and create something beautiful and meaningful to do with the time you have today rather than trying to resurrect and recreate the past. You may find that the things you thought you were afraid of are a blessing if you let yourself stop running the race and sit with you awhile.

✦

I was talking to a friend about how I live my life according to my PET schedule. She told me I was blessed to have a relative idea of how long I was expected to live because it must be "extremely freeing" to plan life without all of the uncertainty. I guess that's one way to look at a five to eight year life expectancy.

I realized that the fear of recurrence I had in regard to making plans was not solely because I feared a second recurrence of cancer, but was in large part because I feared the uncertainty that came with having a life that extended beyond my day planner. Living in six-month increments was safe, it was unburdened, I could be less accountable, take higher risks, and throw out contingency plans. I did not need to eat healthily or go to the gym, I didn't focus on bone health and supplements to counter the debilitating side effects of cancer treatment, because I wouldn't be around to have to put the pieces back together. I could have my cake and eat it too.

✦

The first time that I was became aware of the concept of the new normal. I had no idea what it meant. At first, I did not join any survivor organizations or groups, or take the time to discuss survivorship with a counselor who specialized in the transition period between treatment and life after. I assumed that most everything aside from the physical changes would return to its former state. I believed that what little I had left I could salvage and that if I just tried hard enough that it would all go back to normal. This was an overly simplistic and naïve perspective. As I learned over the two years following my treatment, nothing returned to what it was before I was diagnosed with cancer.

The only thing that has remained relatively the same is the color and texture of my hair. It's as if the rest of me has aged fifty years.

✦

Often cancer survivors experience a sense of melancholy upon learning that they are a cancer "survivor." I believe this comes from two sources.

First, there is no clear finish line. Unlike many other traumas where the event occurs and then it's over, cancer survivors are faced with living with a chronic condition that could turn back to an emergency at any moment. Second, patients may ask the "why me?" question again. However, this time the patient is questioning why he or she has survived as opposed to another patient who may have died.

When I survived, my initial reactions were anger and frustration. I felt a great amount of guilt for those feelings when the "correct feelings" should have been an overabundance of joy and gratitude. I believe this has in part been because I did not fear my own mortality. I never questioned my faith or whether there was life after this one, nor the existence of God.

✦

The bone marrow transplant saved my life and gave me the time I have left. September 3, 2012, I watched the tiny package of stem cells be hooked up to my machine as nurses gathered around my bed with calendars and pony drawings and happy birthday stickers celebrating what they called my new birthday because the transplant changed my DNA. My new DNA even needed new "childhood" vaccines. At that point the only thing I could do was smile because I was choosing the treatment for my loved ones' sake, not my own. I never thought in my wildest dreams that it would work.

When I learned that I was going to survive a little longer, my first reaction was anger. After all, I had just spent such a large portion of my adult life in a hospital bed learning to come to terms with my mortality. When I thought that I was prepared to die and no longer had any need for life, then I had to learn how to live again.

It is very common for patients to go through a stage of depression or anxiety following the completion of cancer treatment. As Dr. Lynn Million, my radiologist at Stanford University Medical Center once told me, "Cancer treatment offers a certain level of comfort" for patients who have been attending treatment monthly, weekly, and even daily. The end of treatment creates a void in the amount of time they spend with their medical teams and doctors. This distance can create anxiety as well as lead to depression.

Many patients feel a sense of being "cut off" from the medical world and are left with much more free time to recover and try to rebuild what they had lost over the course of treatment. This can be overwhelming both physically and psychologically. It is important that there remains a support system during this time, as the patient works to piece their life back together.

✦

*What the hell is it doing? Why is it thrashing its hands around like that? Don't stare—here it comes! Jesus…John…is it…it can't be! Oh good lord I think it is! It's charging right for the…[inaudible]*

　　*Tonight, breaking news out of Palo Alto. An unknown impersonator of Uncle Fester, a classic family spook character from the beloved Addams Family movie saga, has heaved destruction upon the local mall. In a whirlwind display of uncoordinated chaos, which witnesses can only describe as a full frontal assault, Fester has made his descent on a beloved Sprinkles ice cream store.*

　　*Officials have released a statement confirming today's events were a result of his apparent uncontrollable compulsion to thrust his hands, then feet, directly into the vats of delicious Sprinkle's ice cream.*

　　*Wait, I am getting an update—correction, Uncle Fester is in fact not a he but a she, and a cancer patient, and this folks, is neuropathy.*

Neuropathic pain is often described as a burning pain accompanied by tingling or numbness. It may include icy cold or burning hot sensations in various parts of the body. Cancer patients may often find relief in neuropathic or opioid pain medication. Alternatively, cancer patients are often prescribed a variety of different medications "off-label" to deal with the pain. Some examples of these include antidepressant and anticonvulsant medications.

Chemotherapy is often a cause of neuropathic pain. It can be difficult to diagnose due to the fact that the patient may feel pain and weakness from multiple sources, and thus it is hard to distinguish which, if any, is neuropathic pain. It is also exceedingly difficult for physicians to diagnose and treat neuropathic pain in cancer patients due to a lack of comprehensive studies on the subject matter.

# CHAPTER EIGHTEEN

# FIRST COMES LOVE

*Loss of fertility occurs at a high rate in cancer patients, especially those receiving chemotherapy and radiation treatments.*

✦

In 2008, I was going to study economics abroad at Cambridge. I had just finished my political science degree at the University of Nevada, Reno, and was thrilled to be going back to England. It was my second term at Cambridge and that year I would be living on Warkworth Street with eleven other students. I had never lived with people I hadn't known before, let alone eleven of them. The first day I moved into the house, there was a small orientation about the house rules and procedures for the year. Across the room I glimpsed a tall blonde-haired, blue-eyed boy. We were briefly introduced. His name was Harrison Powers, and he was a lacrosse player from Dallas, Texas.

After our first meeting, I was a little intimidated and tried my best to avoid him at all costs. Like everyone else in the house, he was a few years older than me and already seemed perfectly at home in a new country. He was not a person I was interested in because, at the time, I was focused on securing my internship at an economic consulting firm. In fact, he was the last person in the house I eventually got to know. After several weeks had gone by a friend of mine was planning a weekend trip to Belfast and Dublin and invited me along. I managed to get out of work and tagged along for the trip.

The morning we were leaving for Belfast, we had to be up by three am to walk to the bus station. By the time I finished packing my things and got caught up on work for the weekend, I was rushing to leave for the bus. I hurriedly opened my bedroom door and bounded down the stairs, and wound up staring Harrison straight in the face. He was going to Belfast too. During the trip, Harrison and I became close. We talked about our dreams, families, educations, and backgrounds. I decided that my preconceived notions of the lacrosse player from Texas had been skewed and reckless. I had imagined a Republican snob, a stupid jock. But he was open-minded and smart. By the end of the trip, I found that I thought well of Harrison, and we became quick friends, inseparable except at times when we had classes or I had to work.

My traditional idea of a first date is something along these lines: the boy arrives to pick up his date dressed in a casual yet stylish outfit. More times than not, he is wearing too much cologne and his hair is overstyled. He talks in a nervous stream all night long, pivoting from subject to subject trying to fill the silences. The girl wears something more akin to business casual, a step or two more formal than her date, also has overstyled hair and just a little too much makeup. She is nervous and does not say much, except to respond to a few cues and jokes. Dinner is at a restaurant neither of them can really afford, French perhaps, and the conversation is boring—staunchly steering away from non-neutral issues such as politics and religion. Each person, acting on their best behavior, tries to conceal any character flaws. That is what I expected from my first date with Harrison, but Harrison has never been predictable.

It was October 15, 2008, and I had just come home from a long day of work at the firm. It was time for the weekend, and I was happy that most of my other housemates were going out of town, and the house would be peaceful. It was also the weekend Harrison had first asked me out on a real date. As I was deciding what I would wear to one of the handful of restaurants we had been to several times during our friendship, I heard a knock on the door. I opened it; there stood Harrison.

I smiled and said hello but he just looked at me with a smirk and said, "Are you ready to go?"

I was confused since it wasn't Friday—our agreed upon date night—and I thought maybe I had gotten the dates wrong.

"For what?" I said.

He handed me an envelope and said, "Our date tomorrow night. If we don't leave soon, we won't make our reservations, so hurry and pack."

I looked down at the envelope and opened it, and there was a ticket with my name imprinted on it leaving for Geneva, Switzerland, in four hours. I almost died!

We flew into Switzerland and stayed at a beautiful hotel near Lake Geneva. We ate dinner at the Casanova Restaurant. We were the only people there, and the food was delicious as well as the wine. The next day Harrison and I took a train to Interlaken for a night (and, no, I'm not saying whether or not we shared a room), where we went hiking in the Swiss Alps and toured glaciers, some of which had ice works displayed inside of them. When we returned to England, Harrison and I were closer than we had ever been.

Our relationship only progressed after our trip. When our semester at Cambridge was over, we returned to our separate colleges. By then, however, we realized we could no longer live apart, and we moved in together. Our life as a couple took us to San Francisco, Connecticut, and eventually Texas. Our future was limitless. We envisioned booming careers, a lovely home, and, of course, the pitter-patter of little feet.

✦

When I found out I could never have children because of the cancer treatment, I wanted to fall to the ground sick to my stomach. I wanted to scream. I wanted to lash out in a fit of rage. While I know that I would have chosen the same path of treatment that ultimately was selected for me, it was not a decision I made for myself. Therefore, a part of me was still angry and resentful because I had been given no choice. It was a decision that was made for me in spite of my young age and in complete ignorance of my desires to have children of my own.

The aggressive chemotherapy (BEACOPP) was the difference between life and death, but it would make me infertile. Doctors have been known to not tell patients of the destruction of fertility if they feel the patient may choose fertility and having children over having this life-saving treatment. The doctor insisted on the first round of BEACOPP even though she knew my medical team was working on preserving my fertility.

What I'm saying is, I would have chosen the treatment; it was life or death. I would have chosen life. But I was still upset because they didn't give me a chance to choose. They took away my fertility in one fell swoop without any warning at all.

I was informed of my infertility right after my first BEACOPP treatment. My fertility doctor told me. He told me he hadn't known they were going to do the BEACOPP treatment. My blood test after, to tell me how many eggs I had left, came back at 0.16, which is the lowest the test could go, meaning my fertility was near zero. My fertility doctor was upset that the oncologists performed the BEACOPP treatment without his knowledge, knowing they were trying to preserve my fertility from day one. But at that point, there was nothing he could do. We did try the fertility treatment anyway, but it didn't work.

In the end, I wonder if it may have been easier for me if I would have had the option to choose for myself outright. I suppose it's not the ultimate outcome that infuriated me but that another person made the decision for me. My doctors did not disclose any crucial information that would have made it clear that in proceeding with the second chemotherapy regimen that the chances that I would be infertile were close to 100 percent. It only took one treatment cycle of chemotherapy to make me sterile and put me into menopause at the age of twenty-five.

Fertility is one of the most critical issues cancer patients face, particularly young patients. Over the previous decades, fertility issues were not discussed with patients unless the patient brought up the concern. However, loss of fertility occurs at a high rate in cancer patients, especially those receiving chemotherapy and radiation treatments. Today, due to the controversial past of fertility issues in cancer diagnosis, it is crucial that when a patient receives a cancer diagnosis, their physicians discuss whether there is a chance for loss of fertility. Additionally, the physician should discuss with the patient the options of egg freezing and sperm banks in the case that the treatment could result in sterility.

✦

Days like these aren't ones that you typically forget.

I was devastated by the loss of my fertility. Especially knowing the value Harrison placed on family. This was not what he signed up for.

The only thing Harrison ever wanted was a family, a beautiful, comfortable house in a good school district, and a Labrador. I knew I had to tell him that I was not only completely unable to have children but that I also could not carry children because it might result in recurrence. I was so afraid I would lose Harrison that I tried to dump him, to spare him. But after I told him (the same day I found out), he didn't even blink.

He exhaled and said, "Sarah, this is my life, and it's my choice whether or not I want to be with you, I choose you! I choose you, Sarah! No matter what! So we'll adopt. I want to raise children with you."

I realized how foolish I'd been in my moment of despair. Harrison believed in me, and he believed in us.

One day, Harrison and I will go into an absurdly bright and optimistic fertility clinic, with an overly friendly staff, and too many selections of beverages. Harrison will have a Dr. Pepper, and I might just have coffee or tea. We will sit tapping our toes nervously trying to mask the pain behind the reason we are here. I'll take notice of the type of magazines at this fertility clinic: they'll all be motherhood magazines. The covers will feature pregnant women in various poses but always with their hands on their belly and looking down with doe-eyed motherly love. I hate this type of picture. I hate it with every ounce of my spirit. It is so extremely hurtful to sit in the waiting room surrounded by images and decorative nonsense that is supposed to make us feel comforted, but doesn't. If anything it'll make us feel even more out of place.

✦

I find that Halloween is too painful for me. On Halloween, I prefer to work in my office while Harrison hands out the candy to all the children in their costumes who are trick-or-treating. I loved trick-or-treating when I was younger. I like to see what my niece dresses up as every year. That is about as much as I can take. But I just cannot shake this relentless feeling that I'm depriving Harrison of the beautiful life that he should be living with someone who is not ill and has the ability to have children. That is not something that I will ever be able to do.

# CHAPTER NINETEEN

# THE GOOD, THE BAD AND THE BINDING

*The uncertainty of what my future holds is unnerving, but I am determined to buy that wedding dress today.*

✦

Through the diversity of my encounters, I have acquired a better understanding of myself, which has increased my faith in my capabilities when challenges arise. I have gained the understanding that the accumulation of my experience will ultimately provide greater rewards than those I seek for myself and the costs I paid to shoulder them.

I've reached an important and unnerving milestone that typically I would manage by relaxing with a glass of merlot, but this one is different. I have been engaged for a little over a year now. I have enjoyed the idea of a wedding and life beyond cancer. In all honesty, I had struggled to believe wholeheartedly, when I closed my eyes at night, that it was more than just a dream.

I've had my wedding dress waiting to be picked up for ten months, but I could never bring myself to return to the wedding store and take my dress home. Well, today is the morning. The morning I finally go to pick up my wedding dress.

The uncertainty of what my future holds is unnerving, but I am determined to buy that wedding dress today. I'm letting myself start to dream and plan again for a future that does not expire in six months with the next PET scan.

When do we allow ourselves to try to live again? Not just existing as survivors of cancer, but truly living a fulfilling, rich life in the aftermath of all we have experienced. It is much scarier than I imagined it would be, to want more than to just survive, and to make a sincere effort to learn to move beyond treatment. I'm trying to build a life where I am living with cancer instead of under it.

I hope the dress still fits!!

# ACKNOWLEDGMENTS

To my mother, Sue Coffey, who faced cancer head-on and was right by my side every single day. For her, it was never an *I*, or *you*, it was always *we*. Thank you, mom, for being the light of my life, my best friend, and strongest advocate.

To my father, Bill Kugler, who was a pillar of strength and love, who was the anchor in the storm, and the man who kept the foundation from crumbling beneath our feet. It is because of my father that my mother and I were able to dedicate every moment to my care and treatment, without the burden of undue delays because of insurance, bureaucratic disorganization, and the ceaseless paperwork that was always urgent and crucial, which he took care of without fail every single day. Thank you, Dad, for always being ten steps ahead, ensuring that my treatment and care never fell behind.

To Harrison Powers, a remarkable man and the love of my life. I've experienced going around the world and back with you, and I wouldn't have it any other way.

To my sister Alyce Kugler, who has been my champion and greatest ally no matter what the challenge, how difficult, or the sacrifices required. My sister is one of my heroes; her capacity for love and unwavering support is unlike anything else I've ever seen. My younger sister would bear the burden of the world without a second's thought and without any expectations. She would do this purely out of love for me, and has when I was too weak to carry the burdens myself.

To my brother, Morgan Kugler, who alongside my father took on the great responsibility of ensuring that our family and the family businesses remained stable and provided financially during what was an extremely difficult time.

To Allison Kugler, my little sweetie. You'll never know how you helped me get through treatment until you're older, but you helped me tender the storm with a sense of humor and the sweet unadulterated love of a child. Without clean feeties, you can't get in the sheeties.

To my uncle, Richard Coffey, and his family. Richard is an example of a parent who takes opportunities to show and to instill in his children love and compassion for others. I'll never forget his son, Mac, as a young boy holding my hand in the hospital with such love and tenderness.

To the Lowe family, Nancy, aunts Jan and Anne, uncles Tom, Donald, and Kagal: thank you for always having my back. I would like to say thank you particularly to Anne, who made it a point to let me know weekly that she was praying for and thinking of me, by never failing to send me a beautiful card and letter.

To my aunt and uncle Mo and Bob Woodward, who opened their home to me and made it their mission to make sure I was always comfortable, loved, supported, and valued. And also for the pie and the midnight snacks! Even in the darkest of times, you have a special gift for bringing out the light. This is what you did for me, and I can honestly say I look back and smile on those days we spent together despite how ill I was. I remember having fun, and I remember the dinners and the laughter. I remember the love you shared with me and my family, and with me and Harrison. Thank you for such a beautiful gift.

To my aunt and uncle, Mary and Steve Walker, who were unwavering in their support and in abundance of love and strength. It was you both who were there when it really mattered. Amidst all the chaos and the flurry of it all, you were there. And when the dust settled, and we came out of it on the other side, you were there. Steadfast and strong, you were there. A port in a storm, my strength when I was weak. My families rock. I am forever grateful to you from the bottom of my heart, and you both will always be so deeply cherished and loved. Always.

To the Saunders family. Thank you for opening your beautiful home and hearts to me and my family, especially during the time when I was in treatment at Stanford. Knowing that Harrison and my mother had a peaceful, beautiful, calm, loving and serene place to rest while going through such a trying time was an incredible comfort. Thank you Molly for all the times you came and visited me and sat with me day in and day out watching Netflix reruns and *The Real Housewives* mega-empire. You showed me that love comes not only in the grandest of gestures but is felt strongly also in the smallest of kindnesses and actions.

To the Brissenden family, thank you for your support of these past few years and your support for me and this book. You have always been one of the greatest supporters of Harrison and my going after our dreams, especially when it came to taking chances like this one. From the times in San Francisco to where we are now, you have always been there cheering us on.

To Becky Massengill. One of the most supportive individuals during this time was not a family member, but my mother's best friend and a true role model in my own life. Becky and my mother have been friends for forty-five years, and I grew up knowing there was a special bond between the two. Her devotion to others and her strong faith in God drives her to help others in need, and she warmed my heart with the considerate things she continued to do throughout my treatment. Becky was an unwavering support for my mother and me during the most difficult times. Her kindness, strength, her faith in God, and compassion makes me feel blessed that she has been part of our lives. Thank you.

To Tiffany Masten. Thank you for being such a good friend during this writing process. You have been a person who has kept me grounded and honest. You are one of my best friends and one the wisest people I know. I cherish our weekly breakfasts at Angela's Cafe; they are the highlight of my week.

To Paul Green, thank you for being supportive of this project in your own way! You know what I mean.

To Alan Dershowitz. Thank you for sharing your personal story in this book, I know it will touch many lives, as it has touched mine. Thank you for helping me learn to be "unconfirmable."

To Dr. Neil Fiore, you taught me how to mentally and physically approach the long difficult challenge that is cancer, and how to best position myself where I was well informed, and an active participant in my health care, and made the final decisions about my treatment. I have always been sharply aware that there were people who came before me and there would be those who would come after. In sharing your experience with cancer, and the lessons you learned, you have saved at least one life that I know of, and I feel that I have a responsibility now to those who will come after me to empower and encourage them in taking an active role in their health care, in the hopes that they will become their strongest advocate. If

I can impact even just one person in the way your work has impacted me, my experience will not have been in vain and will be worth every single moment. Thank you for the work you have done, and for sharing your knowledge and experiences, which are absolutely invaluable.

To Dr. Ginna Laport, the woman who saved my life in more than one way. Without her expertise and guidance, I would not be where and who I am today. Dr. Laport was the first physician who truly believed in my survival and made my dreams and goals her own in spite of the totality of the circumstances. You always held me to high standards and never once made exceptions for me because I had cancer. I remember in our first meeting, you saw success not only as achieving remission but as getting me back to law school, living a healthy and productive life. Not to mention, everything you have done was accomplished all while wearing beautiful stilettos, taking time to go to the Rose Bowl, plan great family vacations, a smile on your face, makeup done, hair photo ready, and with gumption and sincere compassion for your patients! I am confident you must wear a cape under your lab coat, because apparently Superman is actually "Superwoman," and just so happens to be medical practitioner. Thank you for giving me my life back.

To Dr. Lynn Million, the pinnacle of excellence and devotion to a purpose larger than herself for always holding me as her patient, as well as her colleagues to the highest standards, working with me as a team, and always acting in my best interest without apology.

To Dr. Robert Collins and P.A. Jaime Roman at UT Southwestern Simmons Cancer in Dallas, Texas. These two are the most dedicated team I have ever come across. Thank you for showing me what it truly means to be patient-centered. Thanks for striving for the highest levels of excellence, always seeking to be better than yesterday and for not defining success by measures already in place or in meeting current best practices, but for going beyond and redefying and continuously setting them, and for continuously raising the bar that others measure themselves by. All with great compassion, enthusiasm, and humor. Thank you for treating all aspects of my health and for ensuring that my medical team here in Texas is designed to achieve wellness of my entire person, and for giving all aspects of my health equal weight and importance so that I can truly live a life beyond cancer.

To Dr. Michael Lewandowski. Thank you for being such a wonderful physician and introducing me to Cindie Geddes. You taught me so many valuable life skills and got this project rolling. You were instrumental in bringing this project to life.

To the Stanford Cancer Center and UT Southwestern Simmons Cancer Center, I want to thank the nurses and caregivers who were so kind to me during my cancer treatment. Thank you to the team I entrusted with my life, who fought for me even when it meant going above and beyond their roles in order to ensure that noting and no one compromised my health care and treatment. Thank you to the exemplary physicians who went into medical practice for all the right reasons and always put their patients before themselves.

To Cindie Geddes, the managing editor of this book, who took on this project with a passion and fervor that is rarely seen. Cindie, thank you for your countless nights that you have spent editing and working with me to make this project not just another cancer story, but what we set out for it to truly be. You told me that anyone can write a book that says something, but it is a rare thing to write a book that does something. It is because of you that I believe *we* together have accomplished this. Thank you for helping me take what has been in my life such a difficult experience and turning it into something that I hope will help others. Without you, none of this would have been possible.

To Lucky Bat Books, thank you for taking a chance on a first-time author with a manuscript in one hand and a mission in the other! I am very grateful to everyone at Lucky Bat, all exceptionally talented and kind. You are making the world a better place one story at a time.

To Danielle Tunstall, thank you for designing such a beautiful and gripping book cover. You are a genius! Thank you for standing ground with me and fighting for the cover of this book. It is truly a work of art.

To Sarah Katreen Hoggatt: Thank you for being not only a good friend and spiritual advisor, but excellent at your job. I couldn't have done this without your amazing talents.

To Courtney Sermone. Without her, none of this would have been possible. In what I believe to be a connection divinely ordained, she made me a far better person than I could have ever become alone. She taught me to be curious, to feel the unspoken stories of other people's lives, to not fear the gloriousness of emotion in all of its pain and utter joy. I learned to not just love language, but to find the treasures of story, that is hidden in a language not of words but in between breaths, what we see when we blink, and what our stories tell when words fail us. She made the world a beautiful and colorful place for me where I am once again unafraid to laugh, to cry, and willing to go to the darkest of places with her by my side these last years of my life

I thank God every day for the blessings bestowed on me.

www.ingramcontent.com/pod-product-compliance
Lightning Source LLC
Chambersburg PA
CBHW062056270326
41931CB00013B/3101